Bath Bombs

The Ultimate Guide to Homemade Bath Bombs

(A Well Detailed Guides to Making Bath Bombs for Relaxation)

Rachael Gilbert

Published By **Adan Kalcanto**

Rachael Gilbert

Bath Bombs: The Ultimate Guide to Homemade Bath Bombs (A Well Detailed Guides to Making Bath Bombs for Relaxation)

ISBN 978-1-998769-43-8

Legal & Disclaimer

The information contained in this ebook is not designed to replace or take the place of any form of medicine or professional medical advice. The information in this ebook has been provided for educational & entertainment purposes only.

The information contained in this book has been compiled from sources deemed reliable, and it is accurate to the best of the Author's knowledge; however, the Author cannot guarantee its accuracy and validity and cannot be held liable for any errors or omissions. Changes are periodically made to this book. You must consult your doctor or get professional medical advice before using any of the suggested remedies, techniques, or information in this book.

Upon using the information contained in this book, you agree to hold harmless the Author from and against any damages, costs, and expenses, including any legal fees potentially resulting from the application of any of the information provided by this guide. This disclaimer applies to any damages or injury caused by the use and application, whether directly or indirectly, of any advice or information presented, whether for breach of contract, tort, negligence, personal injury, criminal intent, or under any other cause of action.

You agree to accept all risks of using the information presented inside this book. You need to consult a professional medical practitioner in order to ensure you are both able and healthy enough to participate in this program.

TABLE OF CONTENTS

Part 1

The Making of Bath Bombs In the Nutshell

Bath bombs are made to let a pleasant scent linger and to fill your bath with a bit of sparkle, some color, or perhaps an entire rainbow. While commercial bath bombs can cost around $5 to $15 each homemade and custom bath bombs are much easier to make and less costly and include the ingredients you want to use as well as knowing precisely what goes into making the bombs.

Most bath-bomb recipes contain similar ingredients. Below are the top popular ingredients:

Baking soda

This ingredient that is alkalizes is usually the base of bath bomb recipes. it's job is to produce the highest fizzing reaction. Baking soda is also a great way to neutralize or complement the citric acid, and is typically used in higher amounts than acid.

Citric Acid

It is necessary to include citric acid in baking soda to help in the reaction that causes the fizz. However citric acid might not be readily available in many local stores, however you may be able to find it in winemaking and cordial making industries that make homemade cordials.

Corn Starch or Arrowroot

While corn starch and arrowroot are used to thicken the texture in many recipes, you can use them to create the silky texture that bath bombs provide. While corn starch gives more silky feel than arrowroot, make sure you purchase an organically-made version.

Salts and oils

You are in the position of choosing the best mixture of liquids and salts like water or something organic such as witch hazel that is more relaxing. With regards to the salts, you can pick any of the basic sea salts to the refreshing Epsom salt, which also assists to detoxify. Additionally, you can add handful of common oils like coconut oiland jojoba oil, sweet almond oil and olive oil that can help decrease the amount of essential oils too.

Essential oils

They are a scrumptious, highly concentrated natural compounds that are derived from the flower, the roots and stems, as well as bark and seeds, as well as other plant parts. They are referred to as ethereal oils or volatile oils. They're responsible for the distinct scent of plants. They are used for a variety of purposes which range from helping to treat skin ailments and mental disorders to helping rest or improve sleep, as well as other home-based applications. It is possible to add the essential oils in your bath bombs dependent on the type of bath bomb that you're creating.

These are some of the frequently utilized essential oils:

* Rosemary

* Peppermint

* Orange

* Lime

* Lemon

* Grapefruit

* Ylang-ylang

* Rose

* Lavender

* Jasmine

* Chamomile

As we'll be using essential oils in a few in our dishes it's essential to be aware of what to do with them as they can be extremely volatile.

How to store essential oils

Essential oils are intended to last for 5-10 years. Because they are extremely concentrated, a small amount will last for years. The biggest challenge is that essential oils can be degraded by various elements like direct heat, air, or light. This is why it is important that essential oils are stored in sealed, dark-colored containers or bottles to avoid the direct exposure to environmental conditions. For citrus oils like orange or lemon essential oils, keep them in the refrigerator for 5- 10 degrees Celsius to avoid the oxidation or damage caused by fluctuations in temperature.

Colors

If you're looking to change colors in your bathtub, think about the use of natural dyes, or even some drops of food coloring in liquid form.

Let's now take a look at the equipment you need:

Equipment required

The biscuit cutters are made of plastic an ice tray

- Silicone cupcake cups

* Silicone Ice Cube Trays for Ice

* Easter egg packaging

* Plastic packaging for toys

• Christmas decorations like the star

*Pots of yogurt or pudding

* Mini-muffin Tins

* Candy pans

The best tips to make bath bombs

* Make use of liquid food coloring rather than gels because gels tend to clump together when mixed together with baking soda. It could be difficult to mix them all together.

Once you have added the liquids and everything other ingredients to your bath bomb put the mixture in the mold right away.

* To make sure that your bath bombs remain are dry and uniformly dry, it's recommended to keep them in a dry and

cool location as humid temperatures will slow the process.

If you happen to have a mix of several shades, you can make an ombre-colored bath bomb by layering colors in order to create an amazing mix.

When you're completed with all the necessary ingredients Let's head on to our recipes.

Bath Bombs

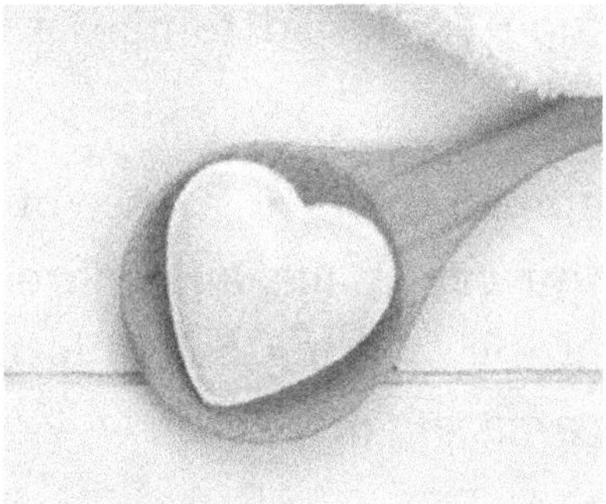

Ingredients

Dried herbs powdered like ginger or 30-40 drops essential oils

1 tablespoon of vanilla extract (or more water)

2 tablespoons witch hazel (or water)

2 tablespoons of the liquid oil you prefer

4 ounces of cornstarch (about 1/4 cup)

1/2 cup (4 ounces) sea salt or Epsom salt

4 ounces of citric acid (1/2 cup)

8 1 ounces baking soda (about 1 cup)

Instructions

1. Then, mix your preferred oil along with essential oils into baking soda. Mix the mixture thoroughly.

2. Add the dry ingredients, which are the citric acid, cornstarch as well as salt. Mix until well-integrated.

3. Then add the powdered ginger or any other herbs you like.

4. Apply the witch hazel spray to the mixture in a very careful manner. It is possible to use spray bottles.

5. Mix the ingredients with your hands. Wear gloves if have hands that are sensitive.

6. Mix until the mixture will stay in your hands when you squeeze it, without breaking. It is possible to add less or more witchhazel until you reach your desired consistency.

7. Pour the batter into muffin tins with grease or other molds that are greased and then press them in with a firm press.

8. Allow it to set for at least 24 hours, or up to the maximum of 48 hours should you wish.

9. If the mixture expands in the beginning then just press it to the mold numerous times to stop it from expanding more when it is drying. It is also possible to use an aluminum mold which is more efficient.

10. After the bath bomb has been dry, take it off the mold and put it in the bag or in an airtight container. Make use of the bath bomb for 14 days after it has been stored.

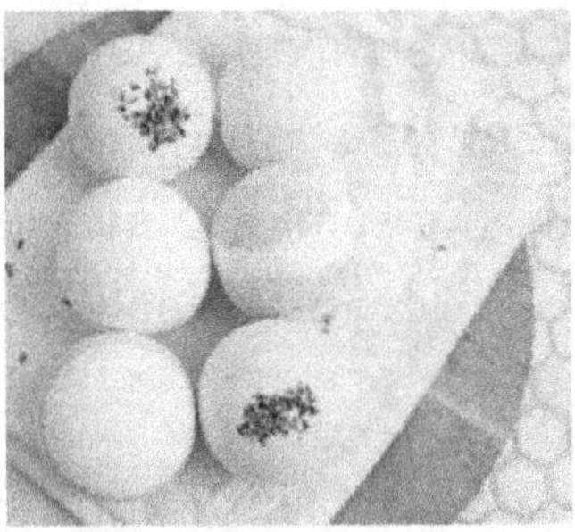

Homemade Bath Bombs

Ingredients

1 1/4 teaspoons of coconut oil or olive oil

5-10 drops essential oil of your choice

1-1/2 teaspoons of water

2 oz. Epsom salt

2 oz. citric acid

2 oz. corn starch

4 oz. baking soda

2 drops food coloring an option

Instructions

1. Mix the corn starchwith baking soda, citric acid along with Epsom salt. Stir the mixture until it is free of any clumps . Set aside.

2. Mix together the liquid ingredients, including water olive oil as well as food color.

3. If you decide to use coconut oil instead the olive oil you must first melt it on your

stove or microwave to aid in making it to blend easily into the mix.

4. The liquid blend should be gently poured to the dry ingredient and mix thoroughly until well-integrated. If the mixture begins to foam or fizzs, it indicates that you have added the liquid mixture too quickly.

5. Once the liquid and dry mixture is combined the mixture, scoop out a small amount of the mixture , and squeeze it into your hands.

6. Make sure the mixture sticks together in a couple of chunks. If the mixture appears to be too powdery to hold together then add a small amount of liquid and stir until it can stay together.

7. If you find it difficult to add liquid you, think about using spray bottles to pour it into slowly, instead of pouring.

8. Then, fill half of the mold using the mix until the container starts to fill up. After that, combine the ingredients and then

gradually remove one end of the bathtub mold.

9. Place the mold for your bath bomb on a tray, and let it to air dry, then take the opposite part of the mold. Then slowly turn the bath bomb to ensure that the portion that isn't covered is facing downwards and then remove its top.

10. Give it another hour or so , and after that, check whether the bath bomb is able to easily be removed from it without breaking.

11. In the event that it cracks If it breaks, put it back in the mold and let it completely dry. Do not keep it in your mold too long, as it will be more difficult to take them out without breaking.

12. If the bath bomb begins to crack at any point in its removal away from the mold, slowly place it back on top of the second half, or remove the entire mixture , and then begin the process of gaining mold.

13. Once you are able to easily remove your bathing bomb, allow it air dry for around 8 hours, or perhaps for a few days.

14. Wrap the bath bomb that is dry in plastic wrap and keep it in a cool area until you're ready to take them out for a bath.

Lavender Bath Bombs

Yields: 7 bath bombs

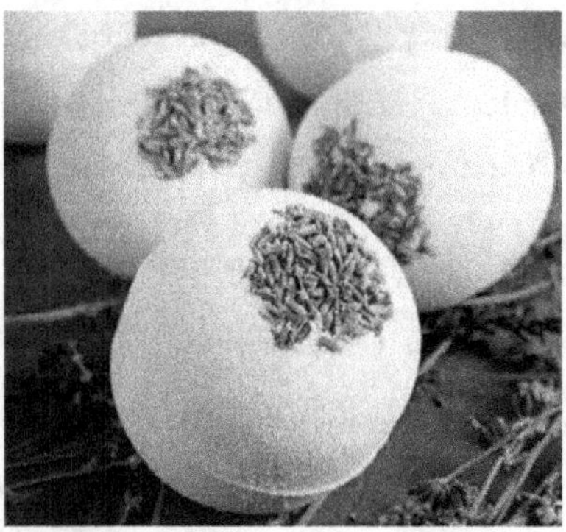

Ingredients

Witch hazel spray bottle

Dried lavender

12 drops lilac la bomb colorant

0.3 oz. lavender essential oil

0.7 oz. polysorbate 80

2 oz. borage oil

4 oz. extra fine Epsom salt

16 oz. citric acid

32 oz. baking soda

Instructions

1. Include borage oil, polysorbate the essential oil of lavender as well as the Lilac La Bomb colorant in the bowl of a small size. Utilize an ice cube to blend the ingredients thoroughly until the mixture is almost all blended but it's still fine.

2. In a large bowl, mix in baking soda and citric acid and break the clumps up with your hands or by pushing the mixture

through the Sifter. It is necessary to wear gloves.

3. Incorporate to the Epsom salt. Stir until the salt is fully incorporated.

4. Incorporate oil into the dry mixture , and mix it all together with your hands. The result should be a wet sand consistency that is held in shape after you press it.

5. If you think the mixture isn't enough moist, add a bit of witch hazel when you mix it with your other hand. Continue to drizzle more water until your mixture is able to hold its shape.

6. Add some dried lavender to the middle of your mold, and then fill both of half of the molds with the lavender mixture.

7. Press the mixture gently in the mold till the mold is full by the contents.

8. Pull the top portion of the mold away while you turn. It can be difficult to make the bath bomb stay together You'll need patience.

9. To take the other part of the mold, put it back in and turn the bath bomb upside down. Then, release the opposite side, twist it, and then pull it off with care.

10. Place the bath bombs in a container that is able to hold the bombs and not roll away , or simply placed on the counter.

11. The bath bombs should be allowed to fully dry, and then harden over the course of a night. If you decide to use the bath bombs, just place them into hot bath water!

Fizzing Bath Bombs

Yields: 16 bath bombs

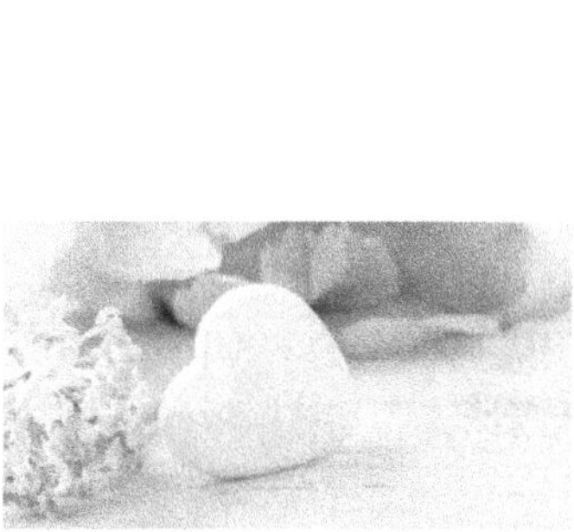

Ingredients

Two teaspoons of witch hazel

5-6 drops essential oil

Three teaspoons of olive oil

1 cup sea salt or Epsom salt

1 cup cornstarch

1 cup citric acid 1 cup

2 cups baking soda

Silicone molds

1 spray bottle empty

Instructions

1. Mix the cornstarch, citric acid baking soda and Epsom salt in large bowl until completely incorporated, without lumps.

2. Mix with olive oil, essential oil. Mix and mix until well-integrated.

3. Spray the mixture with only some witch hazel until it is moist enough to create bath bombs that will be held. Be careful

not to over-moisturize the mix as it could begin to bubble.

4. Place the mix into the molds, and let them rest for 5 or 10 minutes.

5. Take the bath bombs gently from their molds. Then put them on parchment paper to air dry for about 24 hours.

6. To use bath bombs, you just need to add 2 small bombs or one big bomb to your tub and revel in the bubbling effect.

Orange Bath Bomb

Yield: 2 large bath bombs

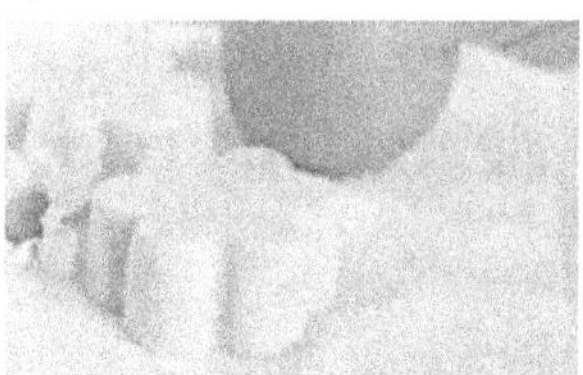

Ingredients

16-20 drops orange essential oil

1/4 cup almond oil or coconut

1 teaspoon zest of orange

1/4 cup Epsom salt

1/2 cup cornstarch

1 cup of citric acid

1 cup baking soda

Water

Food coloring orange, optional

Instructions

1. Within a bowl make a mixture of Epsom salt and corn starch with citric acid, baking soda and. Mix the ingredients until there aren't any lumps.

2. In the microwave, melt some coconut oil your microwave. Once it's melted add the essential oil and food coloring If you'd like.

3. Combine this mixture with mix with the Epsom salt mix and stir thoroughly using your hands.

4. Mix it with a small amount of water several instances until it starts to bind.

5. The mixture should be poured into the mold of your choice, like a plastic Easter egg or plastic ornament mold as well as cute flower molds.

6. Let the bath bombs dry for at least 4 hours before you gently take them out of the molds.

Bathroom Bombs with Orange Crush

Ingredients

1 tablespoon of water

Orange food coloring or gel

1 teaspoon essential oil of orange

2 tablespoons oil of almonds

1/4 cup Epsom salt

1/4 cup corn starch

Half cup acidic citrate

1 cup baking soda

Body glitter, optional

Instructions

1. Mix all dry ingredients with a bowl. place aside.

2. Mix the other ingredients into a tiny mixing bowl. Then mix this mixture to the dry ingredients mix.

3. Mix quickly to stop the liquid from resolving.

4. If there is glitter in your mold, sprinkle it in the molds. Then scoop the glitter mixture inside the mold. Then press it down.

5. Slightly increase the amount of mold, and then press the two halves of the mold together very strongly.

6. Allow the mold of the bath bomb to remain for a few minutes, then take out the other half for speedier evaporate. You can take them out at any time if you want to.

7. The bath bombs should be stored in a cool location in case you'll need them in several days, or place them in a secure container for use over the long-term. This can help keep the fragrance.

Coconut Oil Bath Bombs

Serves as needed

Ingredients

Essential oils that are preferred

Food coloring derived from vegetables

1 teaspoon of almond oil

Three tablespoons of coconut oil divided

1/2 cup Epsom salt

1 cup of corn starch

Half cup acidic citric

1 cup baking soda

Mica Optional

Instructions

1. Mix all dry ingredients together in a large bowl and mix thoroughly. Divide the mixture equally between three bowls.

2. Take one teaspoon of coconut oil into one cup and then let it melt it. Add two to three drops of your favorite food coloring, and stir to mix.

3. Include 1/3 teaspoon of almond oil, and 5-10 drops of the essential oil.

4. Add all the coconut oil mix and color into the bowls that contain dry ingredients.

5. If you'd like to alter the color, melt a bit coconut oil, then add the food coloring. It is then added to the mix and mix.

6. Repeat the process with the food coloring in the two bowls using dry ingredients.

7. Put the mixture in your mold of choice, and then place the colors over each other , and on all sides of the mold.

8. If you are using the ball mold, simply put each of the sides until they are full, then squeeze the sides to form a.

9. Make sure the molds for bath bombs are at a temperature of 20 degrees for 20 minutes.

10. Warm the entire sides of the molds with you hands, which will melt the coconut oil . This will aid in the removal of the bath bomb out of the mold.

11. You can squeeze any side until the bath bomb explodes. The bath bombs can be sprinkled with glitter if would like to add a touch of sparkle.

12. To use bath bombs, add warm water. Then, place them in the tub.

13. The bath bombs will fizze and release their scent, as well as the ingredients to soften the skin. Soak them in water for about 20-30 minutes.

Lemon Bath Bomb

As needed, serve as

Ingredients

Lemon essential oil

2 tablespoons oil of almonds

3/4 teaspoon water

3 tablespoons Epsom salt

1 cup of corn starch

1 cup of citric acid

1 cup baking soda

Food coloring, yellow, optional

Mold for plastic ornaments

Wilton Daisies with icing

Instructions

1. Combine the corn starch and citric acid baking soda, and Epsom salt in the bowl of a large size.

2. Blend the necessary oil with the dye, water, as well as almond oil, in another bowl.

3. Add the mixture of almond oils to the Epsom salt mixture, and stir until it is well-integrated.

4. Check if the mix can hold together by pressing a tiny amount of the mixture together. If it isn't holding it, spray a tiny amount of the mixture with the spray bottle. Don't add too much water to avoid it becoming ruined or floppy.

5. When you've reached the desired consistency, place the bath bomb into the mold you prefer and allow it to dry for a minimum of two hours.

6. Clean it off the mold, and then place the bath bombs on towel to dry, best over night.

Green Tea Bath Bomb

Serves as needed

Ingredients

1/4 teaspoon essential oil of your choice

2 teaspoons water

2 Tablespoons of almond oil

2 tablespoons of green tea powdered

1 cup of corn starch

1/4 cup Epsom salts

Half cup acidic citric

1 cup baking soda

Instructions

1. Combine the corn starch, matcha powder Epsom salt and citric acid into a medium-sized bowl.

2. Mix in the other ingredients and mix thoroughly.

3. Line the cupcake tin or muffin tin with parchment paper , then scoop the batter into the liner.

4. On top, press the mixture with the spoon's back or with your hands. Mix in the rest of the ingredients and push it down. It is possible to smooth the tops for a smooth, even finish.

5. Set your molds into a warm location to air dry for a few hours, or until they're firm enough.

6. You can blow or shake out any remaining crumbs.

Unicorn Bath Bomb

Serves as needed

Ingredients

Lavender essential oil

Cosmetic pigment powder

6 . tablespoons coconut oil melt

6 tablespoons Epsom salt

2 cups baking soda

1 cup citric acid 1 cup

1 cup cornstarch

Witch hazel spray bottle

Instructions

1. Mix together the Epsom salt as well as corn starch and baking soda in one large bowl.

2. The mixture should be divided into three bowls. Add 1 teaspoon of pigment powder of various colors into each bowl. It is possible to add more pigment for a brighter hue.

3. Combine the oil of essential, some coconut oil that is melted, and then divide this mixture among separate bowls. Mix thoroughly until it is well-integrated.

4. Apply a few pumps of witch hazel onto the bowl until it takes its shape.

5. Mix the ingredients in the three bowls to mix in the mold you prefer and let it sit for around 4 hours or, ideally, for a night.

6. Take the bath bombs out gently from the molds , then spray them with ruby

alcohol. Also, sprinkle some cosmetic glitter.

Grapefruit Bath Bomb

Serves as needed

Ingredients

1 teaspoon of water

4 drops grapefruit essential oil

1 teaspoon of beet juice

Three tablespoons of coconut oil melting

2 tablespoons Epsom salt

1 cup of citric acid

1 cup baking soda

Instructions

1. Mix together the Epsom salt as well as citric acid and baking soda into a big bowl, and mix the ingredients thoroughly.

2. Incorporate the oil essential, the juice of beets as well as the coconut oil into the bowl of a small size.

3. Mix this coconut oil-based mixture to the Epsom salt mix until you get the consistency of a crumbly.

4. Check if the mix can be molded into shape and stay put without breaking. If it's too crumbly it's best to add some water for instance, one teaspoon at a time. It must be dry, but flexible enough to form the desired shape.

5. The bath bomb mix should be poured into the mold of your choice, or use an scoops for ice cream.

6. Remove them from the molds and place them onto a baking pan to dry for at least 12 hours or for a minimum of 24 hours.

Lemony Bath Bomb

As needed, serve as

Ingredients

15 drops of essential lemon oil

Tiny spray bottle made of Witch Hazel

Food coloring, soap or yellow dye

3 teaspoons coconut oil melting

3 tablespoons Epsom salt

1 cup of corn starch

1 cup of citric acid

1 cup baking soda

Rose icing decoration

Instructions

1. Combine the Epsom salt with the corn starch and citric acid along with baking soda into one large bowl.

2. Incorporate coconut oil that is melted as well as food coloring and your essential oil. Mix well until it is well-integrated.

3. Then spray a tiny amount of witch hazel until the mixture is able to stay in place when it is pressed to one another.

4. If you notice the mixture crumbling, you can add one to three gentle sprays of witch hazel making sure not to cause any bubbling. The mixture should be lightly moistened but do not soak it in water.

5. Place some rose icing inside the other half of the mold and then push it into your mold.

6. The bath bomb mix should dry until it is dry, or for about 1 hour, then take the mold out.

The relief of Sinus Bath Bomb

As needed, serve as

Ingredients

10 drops lavender essential oil

25 drops eucalyptus essential oil

2 teaspoons oil sweet almond

1/4 cup Epsom salts

1 cup of corn starch

Half cup acidic citric

1 cup baking soda

A blue shower color of a bomb lake

A tiny bit of bath bomb color

Instructions

1. A large mixing bowl mix ingredients of corn starch and citric acid Epsom salt, baking soda. Set aside.

2. Mix together the essential oils of lavender food coloring and eucalyptus essential oils as well as almond oil.

3. Add the essential oil mixture into the dry mix and mix quickly to stop water from re-acting.

4. Make sure you make sure to scoop the mixture into the ready molds and then press the mixture thoroughly inside the mold. It is possible to fill the mold up and then press both molds.

5. Allow the bomb to rest within the mold about a couple of minutes before removing the top portion of the mold in order to let the water evaporate.

6. Take the bath bomb out of the mold and allow it to dry for a while, but ideally over night.

7. Keep the bath bombs in an airtight box or container.

Apple Bath Bomb

Serves as needed

Ingredients

2 teaspoons of apricot oil

2 teaspoons of essential green apple oil

2 teaspoons of water

4 ounces Epsom salts

4 ounces of corn starch

4 8 ounces citric acid

8 ounces baking soda

Instructions

1. A large bowl mix all dry ingredients except for citric acid (corn starch baking soda, baking powder along with Epsom salt).

2. Then , mix Apricot oil essential oiland the water into one small bowl.

3. Incorporate the essential oil mix to the dry mix and mix until the mixture is similar to a wet-sand in consistency.

4. To ensure that the color is uniform, continue mixing and pressing down using spatula the pieces. An even color signifies that the mix is completely integrated.

5. Check if the bath bomb mixture will hold by squeezing a small amount into your fist.

6. Add in the citric acid, and mix it again However, do not mix by hand. Don't add water in the future.

7. The bath bomb mix should be placed in the mold of your choice and let it sit for 15 minutes.

8. Take off from the one end of your bath and let it sit for at least another day or till the ball is set.

9. Add the sticks and leaves after the bath bombs have been completely dry.

Rose Bath Bombs

As needed, serve as

Ingredients

A few drops of witch hazel

6 drops essential essential oil of choice

1 cup sea salt or Epsom salt

2 cups baking soda

1 cup citric acid 1 cup

Food coloring

Instructions

1. Within a bowl mix baking soda and citric acid. Then, mix to Epsom salt, fine grains sea salt. Mix until thoroughly in the.

2. Incorporate dried flower petals, such as dried rose petals to give colour. Alternately, add around 2 drops of food coloring. Mix until well-mixed.

3. Place six drops of your favorite essential oils like mint, rose or lavender in your

Epsom salt mixture, and stir with an wooden spoon.

4. Use a bit of witch hazel from a spray bottle by using one hand, while stirring it using the other hand.

5. You can experiment with different amounts of witch hzel until you reach the desired consistency. Be sure to ensure that the mixture does't get too hot and start to fizz.

6. Scoop the bath bomb mix into the molds you have prepared and let them dry for 5 minutes.

7. Once they are dry, remove these from their mold. Then place them in decorative containers.

Eucalyptus Bath Bombs

As needed, serve as

Ingredients

7-10 drops of essential eucalyptus oil

Food coloring

Spray bottle filled with water

1 cup Epsom salts

2 cups baking soda

1 . 1/4 cup of corn starch

1 cup of crystals of citric acid

Instructions

1. Mix the dry ingredients together in the bowl of a mixer, i.e., Epsom salt, baking soda corn starch as well as citric acid.

2. Add a few drops your preferred color and food coloring. You may also leave out the coloring if you want. Mix until thoroughly combined.

3. Add around 7 to 10 drops the oil from eucalyptus and mix the oil quickly. If you do notice any bubbling, that's normal.

4. At this stage, spray 2 or three times with the water, about 2 teaspoons, or until you've got some form of paste. Start small and stir until your mixture starts to become clumpy.

5. Once the mixture is able to be formed, simply press it into molds of your choice or ice cube traytrays and tightly pack it.

6. After it is firm, flip the mold of the bath bomb over and let the bomb fall to escape. The bath bomb should dry for about 24 hours.

Bath for pain relief Bomb

As needed, serve as

Ingredients

1 teaspoon of fresh rosemary chopped

1 teaspoon peppermint oil 1 teaspoon peppermint

2 Tablespoons Coconut Oil melt

2 Tablespoons of cream tartar

1/3 cup Epsom salts

1/2 cup baking soda

Instructions

1. In a glass bowl of medium size Mix the dry ingredients and chop rosemary.

2. Whisk the ingredients together until mixed, then add coconut oil and peppermint oil.

3. Spray some water using the spray bottle to dampen the mix as the mixture is stirred. The result should be an extremely crumbly mix that will easily hold together when squeezed.

4. Make a scoop of the mixture and place it in ice cube tray and bath bomb moulds using the help of a spoon. Make sure to press it down.

5. The mixture should be sit in a cool, dry location for around 4 hours.

6. Then, you can remove the bath bombs out of their mold and put them in a bath that is warm. Enjoy!

Lemon Bath Fizzies

Ingredients

Witch hazel spray bottle

1 cup baking soda

1 cup of citric acid

Zest of 1 lemon

10 drops lemon essential oil

Instructions

1. Mix the baking soda and citric acid in a bowl, or throw them into the food processor to ensure that the mixture is smooth and well-integrated.

2. Incorporate a couple of drops of the essential lemon oil, and about half of the zest of the lemon.

3. Spray the mixture lightly with witch hazel extremely quickly to make sure all ingredients are well mixed before it starts to fizze.

4. Mix the ingredients with using your fingers until you have a mixture that will remain in place when squeezed between your hands.

5. The bath bomb mix should be pressed into the mold of your choice and silicone cube tray.

6. Make sure to press firmly to fill the molds. Allow them to dry inside Ice cube tray until they are they are hardened.

7. After drying you can scoop them up and place their contents in an airtight storage container until they are ready for bathing.

Star Bath Bombs

As needed, serve as

Ingredients

15-20 drops essential oil

3/4 teaspoon water

2 tablespoons of sweet almond oil

3 tablespoons Epsom salt

1/4 cup corn starch

1 cup of citric acid

1 cup baking soda

Star Wars Death Star mold

Soap colorant or silver dust

Instructions

1. Dust your silver dust in your mold, then put it aside.

2. Mix together the Epsom salt with citrus acid, corn starch as well as baking soda, in the bowl of a large size.

3. It is possible to add a bit of silver pearl dust for some light gray tones in the bathing bombs you use.

4. Combine the oil essential, water as well as almond oil, in the bowl of a small size.

5. Incorporate the oil mix to the Epsom salt mixture, and stir the mixture until it is well-integrated.

6. Take a small amount of the mix to determine whether it holds. If it does not, lightly spray water using the spray bottle every now and then. Don't use a large amount of water because the mixture will not work properly inside the mold.

7. The bath bombs should be pressed into the molds that you already have and let them dry for a few hours.

8. Then you can slowly remove the mold from them before taking them out to bathe in.

Lavender Bath Salt

Yieds 4 (8 oz.) Jars

Ingredients

3 tablespoons of cornflower petals

1 tablespoon dried lavender

2 mg Bulgarian essential lavender oil

3 oz. pink sea salt fine

3 oz. pink sea salt medium

20 oz. Epsom salt, extra fine

Instructions

1. Make a mixture of the Epsom salt and pink sea salt together in large bowls until they are well blended.

2. Incorporate the lavender essential oil and mix thoroughly using your hands.

3. Incorporate the petals of the cornflower and lavender buds, and mix thoroughly.

4. Transfer the bath salts to containers and store the jars in a cold, dry area.

5. For bath salts to be used you just need to add it to hot water bath and then relax!

DIY Bath Salts

Produces 12 pounds

Ingredients

5 - 10 drops essential oil

1 cup of sea salt

1/2 cup baking soda

1 - 2 tablespoons dried spices

1 tablespoon coconut, almond or jojoba oils

Colorant of your choice

1 cup Epsom salt

Instructions

1. Within a large bowl combine all the ingredients above and mix thoroughly until the essential baking soda and oil have completely dissolved.

2. The mixture should be divided among the containers as you would like.

3. It is possible to use the bath salt straight away or store the bath salts in an airtight jar.

4. To add salt, you can add about 1/4-1/2 cup to each bath.

Bubbling Bath Salt

Serves as needed

Ingredients

3 cups Epsom salts

1 cup Rock Salt

Instructions

1. A large mixing bowl is required to mix all the ingredients together until it is well-

mixed. Transfer the mixture to an airtight container.

2. Incorporate 1 - or 2-scoops of bath salt to the bathwater.

3. The bath salt should be stored for no more than 3 months in a dry airtight container.

4. Make sure not to scoop out the bath salt using dirty fingers to prevent contamination.

Peppermint Bath Bombs

Yields: 4 bath bombs

Ingredients

1 1/2 tablespoons maty's Vapor rub

2 Tablespoons Coconut Oil

1/2 cup Epsom salt

1/4 cup corn starch

Half cup acidic citric

1 cup baking soda

mold for bath bombs

Food coloring is not required

Instructions

1. Mix all dry ingredients together in a large bowl. Stir until combined.

2. In small bowl, melt the vapor rub, along with coconut oil. You can also add food coloring, if you want to use.

3. Transfer the vapor rub mix into the bowl with all the ingredients that are dry. Mix the ingredients using your hands, and then try to break up any pieces.

4. If you want to alter the color, melt a bit more coconut oil, then stir into the dye you prefer. Pour the dye mix in and stir until it is incorporated.

5. The bath bomb mix should be poured into molds of your choice. For ball molds, fill the mixture until it is full and then squeeze the two half molds for a tight seal.

6. Make sure the bath bomb is at a temperature of 20 degrees for 20 minutes.

7. Simply warm the sides of the mold with your hands to assist in removing the bath bomb out of the mold after the coconut oil is melted.

8. Then squeeze the other sides to the mold till the bath bomb releases.

Kid-Friendly Bath Bombs

Some bath bombs may not be suitable for children. When creating recipes for bath bombs that are safe for children it is important be sure to make use of only natural ingredients and do not include the use of harsh chemical substances that may be harmful to their delicate and delicate skin. Here are some guidelines for making safe bath bombs for children with regard to the ingredients:

Citric acid

In general the citric acid ingredient is a safe ingredient for children. It is commonly added to sweets or juices as well as sauces designed for children. While most adult-friendly recipes call for 1.5 cups of the acid, you can lower the amount to 1/3 cup due to two reasons. Oneis that it makes your bath bombs gentler and, secondly, the less citric acid will result in less sparkling action. Certain kids are more likely to be scared of excessive fizz and may be scared of bath bombs.

Oils

Oils like coconut oil or olive oil can be safe for children . They are advised as they can keep your skin soft and hydrated. Beware of sweet almond oil since it can cause allergies to nuts.

Essential oils

Essential oils that are gentle suitable for children are lavender and chamomile. Lavender essential oil is a great way to help your child relax and assist in improving sleep thus, it's recommended for bathing at bedtime.

It is best combined with lavender, so think about including one-half of each essential oil to this bathing bomb. It is possible to start with five drops of each oil up to 20 or 10 drops based on the child's age as well as the size of your bath bomb, as well as the size of your bathtub.

But, be sure to be sure to limit to essential oils potent for children, for example:

* Essential oil of rosemary

* Eucalyptus essential oil

For these oils that are strong you might need to dilute them using carrier oils, such as grapeseed and coconut oil.

Epsom salt

Although most bath bomb recipes require use of Epsom salts However, it is important to know that certain children are allergic to it. Hence be sure to research the ingredients prior to making use of it.

Oatmeal

In the case of children oatmeal is suggested as it may help to soothe the skin, especially in the case of children who are itchy.

Bath bomb molds

If you are making bath bombs for toddlers or young children take small molds that will result in less bubbling as well as less garish colors.

To keep that in mind, these kid-friendly dishes are for youto try:

Golden Egg Bath Bombs

As needed, serve as

Ingredients

1 tablespoon of water

1/4 teaspoon essential oil for children safe and child-friendly

2 teaspoons almond or coconut oil

1/4 cup Epsom salts

1/2 cup cornstarch

1 cup of citric acid

1 cup baking soda

Purple gel food coloring

Very fine glitter

1 can of edible gold Color Spray

Small toys that go inside the eggs

Large plastic egg molds/candy holders

Instructions

1. Mix together the Epsom salt baking soda, baking soda, citric acid along with corn starch. Add essential oil and water. Then stir the ingredients as swiftly as you can in order to prevent a reaction.

2. Add the food coloring, and stir it all together, add further purple gel till the bath bomb's mixture is from medium purple to deep purple.

3. The individual sides in the egg candy holders with mix and place a toy on the largest side of the egg.

4. The mixture should be pressed down around the mold and on the other side until the mold is completely filled. Then, add additional mixture.

5. After the sides are filled and the sides are full, simply press down on the bath bomb mix and then put 1 additional scoop to each side, then make sure to press it firmly.

6. Fill the molds with the contents in a cool area for about 30 minutes, and then take them out to let them dry for an hour or longer. Paint the molds.

7. Once the bath bombs have dried then spray them using a bottle of edible gold. You will need several coats to completely cover the molds completely.

8. Sprinkle some cosmetic glitter over the wet mold to give it an additional glimmer.

9. Let the bath bombs dry, best over night Then, keep them within an air-tight container until you are ready to utilize them.

Homemade Bath Bombs

Yields 12-15 bombs

Ingredients

5-10 teaspoons of water

2 tablespoons coconut oil that has been melted or another vegetable oils

4 tablespoons of cream tartar

1/2 cup Epsom salts

1/2 cup cornstarch

1 cup baking soda

Food coloring gel or food coloring

Equipment

Bowl

Cups for measuring

Plastic Easter eggs

Instructions

1. Mix the tartar cream, Epsom salt, corn starch, baking soda and baking powder in the bowl of a.

2. Mix coconut oil and food coloring. Or, if using coloring gel, mix it into the process after the previous step.

3. Incorporate the mixture of coconut oils into your Epsom salt mixture and mix the ingredients until they get a crumbly-like consistency.

4. Make sure you test your hands to determine Make sure the bath bomb will hold up when made.

5. You may add a bit of water, if needed, about 1 teaspoon at a time to stop excessive fizzing.

6. The eggshell mold should be filled up with the bath bomb mix, and then gently press down to allow the mixture to adhere.

7. If children are involved in making the recipe, make sure that the step you are attempting to make is completed correctly, otherwise the bath bombs could be able to fall out when taken out of the mold for eggshells.

8. Make sure to squeeze the mold gently to take your bathing bomb out of the eggshell.

9. It is possible to squeeze and twist the eggshell several times to assist in helping the bath bomb mix to release into the mould.

10. Let the bath bomb rest in a dry towel, preferring over night. It can be used in the tub.

Easy Kids Bath Bombs

As needed, serve as

Ingredients

10 drops lavender essential oil

2 teaspoons of water

2 tablespoons of coconut oil

just a couple of tablespoons of chopped Ivory Original 3 Bar

1/2 cup cornstarch

1/2 cup Epsom salt

1 cup of citric acid

1 cup baking soda

Instructions

1. In a bowl mix corn starch, Epsom salt baking soda, citric acid and the Original Ivory 3-Bar. You can make use of your cheese grater for shredding this Ivory bar.

2. Then mix your essential oils, the melted coconut oil as well as water into an additional bowl. It is possible to place the coconut oil jars over warm water in order to melt it before mixing.

3. Add the coconut oil mix to add it to the Epsom salt mix, but preferably just a few drops at a time.

4. Mix the mixture with your hands until you've created dry, well-mixed mixture that can be held in place easily when rolled , or placed into mold.

5. Transfer the bath bombs into the mold of your choice and let it air dry for about 24 hours.

Kid-Calming Bath Bombs

Serves as needed

Ingredients

20 drops lavender essential oil

1 teaspoon olive oil 1 teaspoon olive

1 cup of citric acid

3/4 cup starch from corn

1/2 cup baking soda

Spray bottle filled with water

Instructions

1. Mix the corn starch, citric acid as well as baking soda into a bowl until thoroughly incorporated.

2. In the dry mix Add essential oils of lavender and olive oil , and mix with your hands until it is well blended.

3. The mixture should be lightly spritzed using the spray bottle until it is able to be easily molded. It is best to do this once or

twice, and mix until the mixture is able to hold well.

4. Put the mixture into your silicone mold of choice and allow it to dry for several hours or, ideally, for a few days.

5. Take the bath bombs out of the molds when they're dry and place they in an airtight jar.

6. To make use of the bath bombs, simply put one of them to warm water, and let your child have fun!

Calming DIY Bath Bombs

As needed, serve as

Ingredients

10 drops of chamomile

10 drops of vetiver

10 drops lavender

1 tablespoon Coconut oil and melt

1/4 cup baking soda

Half cup acidic citric

1/2 cup Epsom salt

1/2 cup cornstarch

Silicone mold

Blue soap colorant

Instructions

1. Blend the baking soda, citric acids Epsom salt as well as coconut oil, corn starch and essential oil until thoroughly well-integrated.

2. You could also add food coloring of your choice or blue soap colorant, if you prefer. Keep adding small amounts at each time until you achieve the desired outcomes.

3. Use a spray bottle to spray a small amount of water onto the bath bomb mix by kneading it with your hands continuously.

4. Make sure that the mix is moist enough to mold, but not wet enough so that it

triggers a fizzing reaction. You can squeeze it after to establish that it is sufficiently damp.

5. Make sure to press the mold firmly with a spoon , making sure that it's completely compacted.

6. Let the bath bombs dry, usually overnight, before you gradually remove them from their molds.

7. Keep the bombs in an airtight container, away from the water until it is time to utilize the bombs.

8. To make use of, add 2 or three bath bombs in warm water, and let your child take a bath.

Oatmeal Bath Bomb

Serves as needed

Ingredients

1 teaspoon Chamomile essential oil

2 tablespoons of coconut oil that has been melted

1/4 cup Epsom salt

Half cup oatmeal ground

1 cup of citric acid

1 cup baking soda

The water in a spray bottle

Food coloring, as needed

Instructions

1. Combine baking soda, citric acid Epsom salt and the oatmeal into a medium bowl, and mix well until the clumps have been broken. Set aside.

2. Add coconut oil as well as the chamomile essential oil into another bowl and mix gently.

3. It is also possible to include food coloring in addition to one teaspoon of water to the oil mixture if you want.

4. Add your oil mix to oatmeal in small portions and mix it until well mixed.

5. If the mix appears to be dry, you can spray some water until it becomes a

smooth consistency that is easy to hold its shape when squeezed with your palm.

6. Fill the mold you prefer and press it down with your fingers.

7. It is now time to take the bombs out of their molds and allow they to cool.

Almond & Lavender Bath Bombs

Serves as needed

Ingredients

1 teaspoon essential oil of lavender

2 tablespoons non-scented sweet almond oil

1/4 cup Pink Himalayan salt

1 cup cream of tartar

1 cup baking soda

Spray bottle filled with water

Food coloring in pink as needed

Instructions

1. Mix the essential oil of lavender along with the almond oil into a tiny container.

2. Mix baking soda and pink salt as well as the cream of tartar together in another bowl.

3. Mix the oil and add it with the baking soda. Add several sprays of water each at each time, and mix it with the hands till you achieve the consistency of a moist sand.

4. It is possible to add pink coloring to your bath bomb or skip the coloring completely.

5. Fill the molds you prefer with the mix and press it down using your fingertips.

6. Take the bath bombs out of their molds, and let them to dry. If a bath ball is stuck in the mold, gently tap on the mold until it releases it.

7. These bath bombs should be utilized before bed to help children relax.

Grapefruit Bath Bomb

As needed, serve as

Ingredients

8 drops grapefruit essential oil

1 tablespoon of Jojoba Oil

1/4 cup Epsom salt

1/4 cup cornstarch

3/4 cup of cream tartar

1/2 cup baking soda

A spray bottle of water

Instructions

1. Combine the Epsom salt and corn starch with the cream of tartar baking soda and in a bowl. Then break any clumps that appear.

2. Incorporate essential grapefruit oil and Jojoba oils and mix well.

3. Spray one or two sprays of water in the mixture, and then stir it using your hands. Put gloves on.

4. You can squeeze the mixture with your hands and check to see whether it is stable.

5. Fill two molds using the bath bomb mix and press them to each other.

6. Take the bombs out of their molds, and allow them to dry.

Bath Bombs for children

Yields 4 bath bombs

Ingredients

1 tablespoon of water

15 drops lavender essential oil

Three tablespoons of coconut oil, melted

1 teaspoon coloring color, in the event of you are using

Half cup acidic citrate

1/2 cup cornstarch

1/2 cup Epsom salt

1 cup baking soda

Instructions

1. Mix the citric acid, corn starch, Epsom salt and baking soda in the bowl of a large size.

2. Sprinkle a teaspoon of coloring pigment on the table and mix it well.

3. Make a mixture of essential oils, water and coconut oil that has been melted in the bowl of a small size.

4. Slowly slowly add the essential oil mix slowly to your Epsom salt mix until integrated. It should result in a wet Sand consistency that is able to hold well.

5. Half of your favorite mold using the bath bomb mixture. Add a toy to the middle.

6. Fill the second half of the mixture and then seal both molds. Apply pressure to the bath bombs to seal.

7. Place the bath bomb. Repeat with the remaining three bombs.

8. Let the bombs be set for around 24 hours, then take they from mold.

9. Store them in a glass container that is airtight for no more than six months.

Easy Bath Bomb Recipe for Kids

As needed, serve as

Ingredients

10 drops of essential oil Lavender

Natural food coloring, or water-soluble soap dye

1 tablespoon coconut oil melted.

3 Tablespoons cornstarch

12 cup citric acid

1 cup baking soda

Water to spray

Extras

1/4 cup Epsom salts

1/4 cup colloidal oatmeal

Instructions

1. Mix corn starch with baking soda in the bowl of a large one until it is incorporated.

2. Add a couple of drops of soap coloring, and sprinkle a bit of warm water over it to make the color mix better. Mix thoroughly.

3. Mix until you've got the same shade. Continue adding drops to color until you have the color you prefer.

4. Blend the essential oil with coconut oil in a different bowl.

5. Pour your essential oil mix into the bottle along with baking soda, and mix using your hands and gloves or by using an electric whisk.

6. Mix until you have an emulsified consistency that isn't damp. If the mix is extremely heavy and wet wait for it to dry for a couple of minutes.

7. Add the citric acid, and mix until it is blended. The result should be a mixture that appears as if it is wet sand.

8. Check if the mix can be held together when squeezed into your palm. If it isn't you, spray it with the mixture with 1 to 2 sprays.

9. Make sure to pack the bath bombs into the mold of your choice and press using your fingers until it is tightly sealed.

10. Allow the mixture to rest inside the mold for couple of minutes, then take it out to air dry for around 24 hours.

11. The bath bombs should be stored within an airtight bag until they are ready to use.

Citric Acid Free Bath Bombs

As needed, serve as

Ingredients

2 cups baking soda

1 cup tartar cream

1 tablespoon olive oil

Dried lavender, if needed

10 drops Lavender essential oil

Food coloring

Ice cube traytrays

A spray bottle of water

Instructions

1. Mix the essential oils, olive oil baking soda with food color until you have the desired color.

2. Infuse up to 3 or 2 sprays, and rapidly mix it with your hands until it begins to bubble until you have the consistency of wet sand.

3. Examine if the mixture is able to stay the shape you want by making indentions using the spoon. It should be able to leave a nice form without breaking.

4. Transfer the bath bomb mix into ice cube tray. You could add a few additional sprays of water if required.

5. Incorporate just a small amount of dried lavender, and then fill the silicone or ice cube tray. Make sure to press the mixture firmly to ensure that it's fully packed.

6. Let the mixture dry for approximately 1 or 2 days.

7. Remove the bath bombs slowly from the molds before using them in the bath.

8. If bath bombs fail to break after removing them from the mold simply crumble them once more and spray them with a small amount of water and then return to the molds.

Basic Bath Bomb Recipe

Gives 4 half-balls

Ingredients

1 teaspoon of essential oils like chamomile or lavender

2 tablespoons coconut, sunflower or olive oil

25g cornflour

50g citric acid

100g of bicarbonate soda

A couple of drops of food liquid coloring

25g Epsom salt, optional

The petals of roses, the orange peels or lavender for decoration, optional

Instructions

1. Put all of the Epsom salt, cornflour citric acid , and bicarbonate in a container. then mix them until they are well-integrated.

2. In a small bowl include the essential oil in the form of sunflower oil, as well as the food coloring. Mix well until well mixed.

3. In a gentle manner, add your essential oils and the food coloring mix to your dry

food ingredients, in small batches and whisk them after each addition.

4. After you've added all of the oil then add the water in a couple of drops and then whisk it for a second time. Mix it fast as it will begin to bubble when you add the water.

5. The mixture should form a clump when you press it with your fingers and keep its shape, so make sure it doesn't get wet.

6. If you'd like to add flower petals or some peeled pieces to embellish you can drop them in the top inside the mold.

7. The bath bombs should be pressed carefully on top of decorations, then press down. Use a teaspoon to smooth the bath bomb mixture over.

8. Allow the bath bomb to remain within the mould for around 2 - 4 hours, and then gently take it out of the mold. Then, you can put it in your bath!

Pink Bath Bomb

As needed, serve as

Ingredients

3 tablespoons olive oil

2 . teaspoon essential oil

1 teaspoon of water

1/2 cup Epsom salts

1 cup of citric acid

1 cup baking soda

Food coloring that is red

Instructions

1. Place the dry ingredients in an unmixed bowl. Mix with the whisk.

2. Mix the other liquid ingredients into a different container. It is also recommended to add essential oils, fragrances and the colors.

3. Add the liquid mix into the dry ingredient in tiny quantities.

4. Once the mixture has been thoroughly blended and compacted, place the mixture into a mold , and let it dry. Make sure to work quickly to ensure that the mix doesn't dry out prior to inserting it into the mold.

5. You can also make the bath bomb shape with your hands in shapes like snowballs.

DIY Bath Bombs

Yields 4 bath bombs

Ingredients

12 drops essential oil

3/4 teaspoon water

2 1/2 tablespoons of melted almond or coconut oil

1/2 cup cornstarch

1/2 cup Epsom salt

1 cup of citric acid

1 cup baking soda

Coloring pigments - available

Instructions

1. Blend all ingredients together in the bowl of a medium size and add a small of color, based on the look you prefer. Stir until the ingredients are well mixed.

2. Combine the dry ingredients together in another small bowl until they are incorporated.

3. Mix the wet ingredients in the dry ingredients very gently to ensure that you don't trigger the reaction between baking soda and citric acid.

4. Mix the ingredients together to create a moist and sad consistency.

5. Now, you can fill every mold half with the mixture, then pack it little until it is overflowing. After that, press the two halves quite firm.

6. Let the filled mold rest for about one minute, then gently tap it and gently empty it from the bathtub bomb.

Let the bath bombs dry for at least 24 hours prior to using them in the bath.

Bath Bomb Recipe

Serves: As required

Ingredients

2 teaspoons oil

Two teaspoons of essential oils

3/4 teaspoon water

1/2 cup cornstarch

1/2 cup Epsom salt

Half cup acidic citric

1 cup baking soda

A couple of drops of food coloring

Flowers that have dried or sugar cake decorations Optional

Instructions

1. In an enormous mixing bowl, mix all the wet ingredients together and then transfer

the mixture to an jar that has a top. Then, close the jar and shake it thoroughly.

2. Mix all the dry ingredients together in a bowl, excluding citric acid. Put the liquid mix into the bowl with the dry ingredients , and mix thoroughly with your hands.

3. Add the citric acid, mixing until you achieve a wet beach sand texture. Don't add water.

4. The mixture should be packed very tightly into molds of your choice. It is possible to fill the molds up and then press the mixture tightly over the top with the spoon.

5. After they have been set, remove the bath bombs from their molds and place them on a waxed paper. Let them dry, best over the course of a night.

6. Let the bath bombs dry completely within one to two days before you begin using them. You can simply put them into the tub and revel in the bubbly and flash of color while you inhale the fragrance.

Lush Bath Bombs

Serves: 10 bath bombs

Ingredients

Dry Ingredients:

4 tablespoons tartar cream

1/2 cup coarse sea salt

1/2 cup cornstarch

1 cup baking soda

A few drops of food coloring, or any shade you like

1 tablespoon of water

Two tablespoons of flavor extract e.g. coconut and almond, or cherry and banana

Three tablespoons coconut oil warmed

Molds made of plastic

Instructions

1. Mix the tartar cream along with coarse salt as well as corn starch and baking soda in an enormous bowl.

2. In the bowl of a small size, pour in coconut oil, water food coloring, coconut oil, and the flavor you prefer.

3. Make sure you pour and stir in the mixture of coconut oil and cornstarch mixture.

4. After it has been thoroughly blended, apply it with a firm press into the mold you prefer and place them on large cookie sheets for drying.

5. If the mix is crumbling as you turn the molds, just add a tiny amount of water.

6. Let the bath bombs dry for at least 24 hours. You can then enjoy them in a warm bath!

Bath Bombs made with Oatmeal and Lavender

Serves as needed

Ingredients

14 teaspoon essential oil of lavender

1 and 1/2 teaspoons of coconut oil

1/2 cup quick cook oats

1/4 cup Epsom salts

1/2 cup cornstarch

Half cup acidic citric

1 cup baking soda

Purple gel food coloring

Instructions

1. Within a large bowl mix together Epsom salt as well as citric acid, baking soda, corn starch and the oatmeal.

2. Incorporate the essential coconut oil, oil of coconut, as well as the food coloring gel. Mix well. Don't add water unless it essential to avoid an allergic reaction.

3. Scoop out a small amount of the bath bomb mix to squeeze. If it seems to be clumping tightly, it means that it's thoroughly saturated.

4. Then, sprinkle lavender flowers over one side of the mold you prefer and then

cover your flowers with bath bombs. Then press it down hard.

5. Make sure to fill the other side, and press down firmly on the mixture.

6. If you're using metal sphere molds, simply bend it gently while you press to make the excess mixture to fall in the bowl help facilitate an easy release.

7. You can then take your bath bombs out of the molds gradually and allow they to cool.

8. Keep the bath bombs in airtight containers , or alternatively in bags that are shrink-wrapped.

Glittery Bath Bomb

Serves: As required

Ingredients

A few drops are the preferred essential oil

1 teaspoon of almond oil

3 teaspoons of water

4 oz. of Epsom salt

4 oz. of cornstarch

4 oz. of citric acid

8 oz. of baking soda

Non-toxic Glitter

A couple of drops of food coloring

Two bowls: one largeand one smaller

Instructions

1. A large mixing bowl combine the dry ingredients and put aside.

2. In a separate bowl, mix all wet ingredients with food coloring. If you'd like color-coated bath bombs simply break the recipe into different bowls.

3. Simply add the wet ingredients to your Epsom salt mixture making sure the mixture does not react.

4. Mix the ingredients using your hands or alternatively with the aid of a whisk until you get the consistency of wet sand.

5. To determine if the mix is able to hold its shape simply pinch it between your fingers. If it sticks, it's a good idea to use. If you feel it's too dry, add some drops of water gradually until you attain your desired consistency.

6. If you'd like to put glitter, you can simply put some in the bottom of your favorite mold.

7. The mixture should be tightly packed into the mold and let it dry at least for a few hours.

8. You can put an uncooked cookie sheet over the mold to keep it small. The bath bombs you have dried inside an airtight container till needed.

DIY Bath Bombs

Yields: 3 bath bombs

Ingredients

1 tablespoon coconut oil

Two teaspoons of essential oils

3/4 teaspoon water

1/2 cup Epsom salt

1 cup of corn starch

1 cup of citric acid

1 cup baking soda

Food coloring, if required

Instructions

1. Mix the baking soda, citric acid, Epsom salt, and cornstarch together in a large bowl.

2. Mix coconut oil, the oil you prefer to use, essential oil and water and food coloring, if you wish to use until thoroughly blended.

3. Mix the essential oil mixture to your Epsom salt mixture, and mix it well until you achieve a dry consistency that can be moulded and shaped when squeezed with hands.

4. To make bath bombs, you need to fill one-half your mold of choice, then fill the rest of the mold.

5. Then add more mix into the second part to the point that it's overflows. Then press two mold halves together , and squeeze for one or two minutes.

6. Unlock your mold and place the bath bombs on an oversized towel.

7. If the bathing bomb doesn't out of the mold as a single ball, you'll have to add water perhaps one teaspoon at a time until you reach the perfect consistency that holds it in the mold.

8. Once you've made your bath bombs place your bath bombs onto a baking pan to dry, and then set for about 24 hours.

9. Now you can make use of the bath bombs, or rather transfer them into an air-tight bottle.

Other Bath Products

Anti-Inflammatory Bath Tea

Foodservice: as needed

Ingredients

1-quart of water

2 cups Epsom salts

1/3 oz. dried yarrow

1/3 oz. dried sweet birch bark

1/3 oz. dried ginger

Instructions

1. Make sure to add water to a pot on the stove, and add the ginger and birch bark.
2. Let the mixture come to a simmer and then reduce the heat to an almost simmer.
3. Add the dried yarrow, and cook for about ten minutes.
4. Then, strain the liquid using a cheesecloth, tea strainer or even a piece old cloth.

5. Incorporate the tea directly into the warm bath, along with Epsom salt.

6. Relax in the tub and enjoy the therapeutic bath.

Sensitive Skin Bubble Bath

Yield 12 Ounces

Ingredients

15 drops frankincense essential oil

20 drops lavender essential oil

1/4 cup chamomile tea , or 10 drops of essential oil of chamomile

1 teaspoon raw honey

1 tablespoon Vitamin E oil

2 tablespoons aloe vera gel

1 cup body wash for sensitive skin

Instructions

1. Mix everything together in the bowl of a small one.

2. Mix the ingredients slowly using a spoon until all the ingredients are completely integrated.

3. It is possible to slowly fold the tea in to decrease the number of bubbles you want to make if you're interested.

4. Transfer the mix to the glass bottle that has the lid.

Moisturizing Shower Gel

8 baths, 8 servings

Ingredients

10 drops lavender essential oil

1 cup of warm water, Distilled water

1/3 cup of castile soap

1 teaspoon 1 teaspoon of xanthan gum

1 tablespoon vegetable glycerin

2 tablespoons of jojoba oil

2 Tablespoons of shea butter melting

Instructions

1. Find a medium-sized bowl and then add the Jojoba oil, the melted shea butter and Glycerin. Sprinkle a small amount of xanthan gum over the entire mixture.

2. Allow the mixture to rest for about an hour or so or xanthan gum dissolves into the liquid mix.

3. Utilize an immersion blender, and blend for one minutes or so until xanthan gum is completely integrated in the fluid.

4. Then add warm water as well as the soap made from castile into the bowl.

5. The soap mixture is then pulsing with an blender for an extra one or 2 minutes, until you've got the consistency of a cream lotion.

6. Pour the shower gel mix into the soap dispenser and make use of it within a couple of days. Shake the container every time before using.

Coconut Body Wash

Foodservice: as needed

Ingredients

10 drops of grapefruit or lemon essential oil

10 drops sweet orange essential oil

15 drops eucalyptus essential oil

1 teaspoon vitamin E

1/2 cup liquid castile soap

1/4 cup raw honey

1 cup of coconut oil

Instructions

1. Place the coconut oil into an oven-safe container and heat it up in the microwave using a moderate heat for approximately thirty seconds, or till it is melted.

2. Include Vitamin E, essential oil as well as honey, and mix the ingredients.

3. Make sure to add the castile soap and mix slowly to ensure that you don't to produce any suds.

4. Move the cleanser for your body into an glass or plastic bottle until you are ready to use it. Be sure to shake the bottle before applying it.

Homemade Shower Gel

Yield: 500ml

Ingredients

60-80 drops essential oil if needed

Organic castile soap 500ml

One cup hot water

Fine salt, 3 tablespoons

Distilled/cooled water that has been boiled as required

Instructions

1. Stir in salt, then add boiling water to it., and let the mixture cool.

2. Put the castile soap into an empty bowl. Add essential oils. Mix well until blended.

If you'd like to dilute the soap, simply add some water distilled in equal amounts.

3. Then, add your salt-based soap mix using a dropper. Ensure that you stir it slowly with each step.

4. Continue adding salty water until you have reached the thickness you prefer. The mixture shouldn't be overly thick, as it may not pass through your lotion pump. Make sure to add some water distilled to make it thinner.

5. When you have achieved the perfect consistency you can transfer the mixture into the pump bottle by using an funnel.

6. If the gel mix becomes clear and bubbly while mixing, let it rest for 12 to 24 hours.

DIY Shower Gel

Foodservice: as needed

Ingredients

2 teaspoons vegetable Glycerin

Five drops Idaho Blue Spruce essential oil

10 drops Ylang Ylang essential oil

1 teaspoon Jojoba oil

One teaspoon of vitamin E oil

1 tablespoon raw honey

1/3 cup castile soap

Instructions

1. Put all the ingredients into an unbeatable bowl. Whisk until the ingredients are well blended.

2. A mason jar filled with the mixture , and cover with a lid for a soap dispenser.

3. Enjoy your well-scented shower gel.

Calming Bubble Bath

Serves: As required

Ingredients

15-20 drops lavender essential oil

1 tablespoon of distilled water

1/3 cup vegetable glycerin

1 cup soap castile non-scented

Instructions

1. In a container, pour in the water, vegetable glycerin and the soap castile.

2. Include your favorite essential oils, such as the relaxing and soothing lavender oil.

3. Then stir it well and transfer it gently into the soap bottle or other container.

4. To take a bath in the bubble you just need to add one cup mix to warm water and then relax in the tub.

5. Be aware that the bubbles won't last as long as commercial bubble baths, however the benefits of lavender grown organically and glycerin can go a far.

DIY Bubble Bath Gel

Foodservice: as needed

Ingredients

1 teaspoon of unflavored gelatin powdered

8 drops lemon verbena essential oil

Two teaspoons of witch hazel

1 tablespoon dried sweet wood-ruff

2 tablespoons vegetable 2 tablespoons glycerin

5 tablespoons liquid castile soap

1 tablespoon dried comfrey

1 tablespoon dried peppermint

2 tablespoons of dried lemon verbena leaves

1 cup boiling water 1 cup boiling

Instructions

1. Then, you should steep citrus verbena, comfrey peppermint, and sweet wood-ruff for around 20 minutes. Clean and dispose of all utilized herbs.

2. Then mix your witch hazel with glycerin essential oil and casting soap together in the small container.

3. Mix the ingredients together and add it to the herbal infusion of lemon. Stir in gelatin until it is fully dissolved.

4. When cool enough to handle, put the bath gel to an unclean jar, or squeeze it into bottles.

5. To make use of the gel to use it, simply add 1 - 2 teaspoons to an unheated bath. You can use distilled water in instead the hard water.

DIY Bath Tea

Yields: 3-5 pouches

Ingredients

1/2 cup dried chamomile

1/2 cup dried lavender buds

5 drops Rose essential oil

10 drops German Chamomile essential oil

10 drops Lavender essential oil

1/2 cup coarse Himalayan salt

1/2 cup Epsom salt

1/2 cup dried rose petals

1 cup of whole dried oatmeal

Instructions

1. Blend the oats in a food processor or blender for approximately 30 seconds or until you have the fine powder.

2. Mix essential oils along with salt, dried flower petals and the powdered oatmeal in the bowl.

3. Put the mixture in pouches and fill them with a less than halfway.

4. The bath tea should be stored in a dry, cool location for no more than 3 months.

5. To drink this bathing tea simply place a bag over the sprout, while the bathtub is filling up with boiling hot water.

6. When the tub is filled take the pouch out and let it float in the tub for a while to get soaked in the water.

7. Then, you can relax in the bathtub and soak in the tub.

Soothing Bath Tea

Foodservice: as needed

Ingredients

One cup tea of the green variety

Twelve drops of essential oils you prefer

1/4 cup dried rosemary

1/4 cup dried chamomile flowers

1/4 cup dried rose petals

1/2 cup Epsom salt

1/4 cup dried lavender

Half Cup Tasmanian sea salt

1/4 cup dried calendula flowers

Instructions

1. Place everything in an empty glass bowl and gently mix it all together like you were making a salad.

2. Place the mix in the mason jar of your choice and seal it.

3. The mixture should be kept in a dry, cool location far from direct sunlight for no more than 6 months.

4. To make bath tea, simply add some tablespoons of it into the center of an muslin cloth, and then tie with twine to secure.

5. Fill your tub with warm water, then place the tea bag in the tub.

6. Relax and soak. When you're done bathing, you can take the herbs out and save the bag of muslin for the next time.

Herbal Bath Tea

Serves: As required

Ingredients

1 cup dried, peppermint leaves

1 tablespoon dried chamomile flowers

1 tablespoon dried lavender flowers

Instructions

1. Place about three tablespoons of dried herb in the pouch of a cotton muslin or an old t-shirt or a sock. put the cloth in a knot to make an Sachet.

2. Attach the loosely tied or hung bag under your tub's spout to allow the water to flow through when it fills up your bathtub.

3. Once the bathtub is full, let the bags to remain in the tub for a while. It is possible to squeeze the bag several times as you bathe and observe whether the bath water alters the color.

4. The herbs should be discarded after you have taken bath, clean and dry the bag to be reused for the next time.

Bubble Bath that includes Lavender

Yields Six (2-ounce) bottles

Ingredients

Rosemary, lavenderand orange and frankincense essential oils

Water

4 oz. bottle of vegetable Glycerin

8 oz. bottle of soap that is unscented

Instructions

1. Pour the castile soap in a bowl, 2 tablespoons of water and 4 tablespoons of vegetable Glycerin. Mix until it is well-mixed.

2. Fill the bottles with soap.

3. Add fifteen drops from your favorite essential oils, such as lavender or eucalyptus. Shake until the blend is smooth.

4. It is recommended to avoid essential oils like lemongrass, thyme and peppermint. Also, avoid cinnamon bark or

leaf bay, and clove as these oils may irritate mucous membranes within the body.

Natural Body Wash

Foodservice: as needed

Ingredients

Essential oil with 10 drops.

2 tablespoons of olive oil, and 2 tablespoons castor oil

Three tablespoons of raw honey

3 tablespoons liquid castile soap

Instructions

1. Slowly mix all the ingredients in a glass measuring cup with the spoon. Mixing with the aid of a hand mixer, blender or a whisk to avoid creating bubbles which cause it to be difficult to transfer the mixture into containers.

1. Put the bathing solution in the glass container and use as you need it. You can

store it for up to a month at the room temperature.

2. While bathing you can use natural sea sponges to make it easier to apply.

DIY Body Wash

Foodservice: as needed

Ingredients

10 drops either peppermint, lavender or eucalyptus essential oils

3 tablespoons of Fractionated Coconut Oil

4 tablespoons vegetable Glycerin

1 cup castile soap that is unscented.

8 Ounces glass pump bottle

Instructions

1. Mix all ingredients in a glass bottle, shake and shake until it is well mixed.

2. Shake the bottle every time before you use it.

Lavender Milk Bath

Serves: As required

Ingredients

1 1/2 cups whole milk powdered

15-20 drops lavender essential oil

1/2 cup baking soda

Instructions

1. Combine baking soda and essential oils in the bowl of a mixer.

2. Once the milk is fully incorporated, mix the powdered milk, and combine thoroughly.

3. The bathing milk should be transferred to an airtight container, and then store it in a sealed container.

4. For use, scoop 1 to 1/2 cups of bath milk or 1/2 cup of bath milk for each usage.

Soothing Milk Bath

Serves: As required

Ingredients

1/4 cup baking soda

1/2 cup Epsom salts

2 cups of powdered milk

1/2 cup of oats

20 drops of lavender essential oil, If you require it

Instructions

1. Add the oats to blender and blend until they're thoroughly ground.

2. Add the rest of the dry ingredients into the mixing bowl along with the oats that have been finely ground.

3. Mix the mixture well to break up any lumps.

4. Put the bath of milk into glass jar that has lid and use it within a couple of days.

A Milk Bath with roses

Yield 10 Ounces

Ingredients

5-7 drops Rose essential oil

2-3 drops of red food coloring is an option

1/4 cup Dried rose petals

1/2 cup Epsom salt

1 1/2 cups of powdered milk, full fat

Instructions

1. Blend the Epsom salt with the powdered milk. Then, add two to three drops of red color.

2. Blend the mixture until get the same color. It is possible to skip the colorants if you prefer.

3. Add the rose petals and up to 5-7 drops of your chosen essential oil. Pick between lavender, chamomile or rose essential oils.

4. Pour the bathing liquid into a sachet, or bottle to store until you need it.

Sea Salt Scrub

Serves: As required

Ingredients

1/2 cup of oil of your preference

Half cup salt from the sea

Essential oils of the preferred choice in the event of a need

Instructions

1. Mix your oil of choice as well as sea salt into a bowl. Mix well until the ingredients are well incorporated.
2. Pour the body scrub into the container.

Sugar Body Scrub

Yield 1 cup

Ingredients

Three tablespoons of extra-virgin olive oil

1 cup pure brown sugar or pure organic sugar

Optional

A few drops of lavender, grapefruit or spearmint essential oils

1/2 small lemon juiced

A few drops of Vitamin E oil

1 tablespoon vanilla extract with no alcohol

Instructions

1. Mix sugar and olive oil together.

2. For this sugar scrub you must first wipe clean your face after showering, and then rub it gently across your body. Rinse it off well.

3. Take a bath for at least 20 minutes to relax your skin. This will assist in making the surface soft and soft.

4. Make sure you apply the sugar scrub 2 to 4 times per week. The sugar scrub must be utilized in the first 30 days.

Brown Coconut Oil and Sugar Scrub

Yield 1 1/2 cups

Ingredients

1 cup of solid (but very soft) coconut oil

2 cups of brown sugar

Extra additions

Essential oils of the top choice

Vanilla extract

Instructions

1. Whip the coconut oil solid as well as sugar and other favorite ad-dons until it becomes the creamy and soft cookie dough.

2. Try using a food processor for only several seconds to stop melts of coconut oil, and to keep the sugar scrub different.

3. If the body scrub splits at any point, store it frozen for few minutes before mixing it.

4. The scrub can be stored within an airtight container a few weeks.

5. To apply, mix the brown sugar body scrub using your fingertips.

Poppy Seed Bath Melts

Serves: As required

Ingredients

15 drops grapefruit essential oil

15 drops lemon essential oil

15g jojoba oil

15g of shea butter

30g cocoa butter

30g of beeswax

Sprinkle of poppy seeds optional

A small silicone mold made of silicone.

Instructions

1. Place the shea butter, cocoa butter, as well as beeswax inside the jar of glass and allow it to cool in a pot along with water.

2. Turn the heat up to medium so that it melts the mixture in the jar.

3. Once it is melted, add Jojoba oil into the melted ingredients and mix. Incorporate 15 drops of each of the essential grapefruit and lemon oils.

4. Sprinkle poppy seeds on the bottom of the mold if you prefer.

5. Transfer this hot mix into the molds, and allow it to cool for couple of minutes.

6. Place the bath melts in the fridge or freezer and let them completely set.

7. Once the mold is set, take the bath melts out of your mold and put the melts in glass jars that have lids.

Coconut Oil Bath Melts

Serves: As required

Ingredients

15 drops lavender essential oils

1 cup of coconut oil, or shea butter and coconut oil

The Ice Cube Trays and Molds

Instructions

1. Then, heat the coconut oil using a large bowl by heating it in your microwave, until

coconut oil is completely melted, which can take anywhere from between 1 and 2 minutes.

2. When it is melted, you can add the essential oils of lavender.

3. Blend until it is well-mixed, then pour the coconut oil into the desired molds.

4. Let the bath melts be cooled down, or store in the refrigerator for just a few minutes.

5. When they are cool enough, take the bath melts out of their molds and place the bath melts in an airtight jar in an air-conditioned, dry area.

6. If your home is hot or temperatures rise to 70 degrees or more it is necessary to keep your bath melts inside the refrigerator to stop the melts from melting.

7. Take extra precautions as coconut oil can cause your bathtub to become slippery, and it could cause you to slide and then fall.

Honey Lavender Bath Melts

Yields 15

Ingredients

30 drops lavender essential oil

1 teaspoon of lavender flowers

1 teaspoon organic stress relief tea

50 grams cocoa butter

50 grams of shea butter

Silicone heart mold

Instructions

1. Make the butters melt in a double boiler or microwave until completely melting.

2. Tea bags. Open one tea bag and then measure 1/4 teaspoon of the herb out of the bags.

3. Add the lavender and tea to the shea and cocoa butters and mix until it is incorporated.

4. Set the silicone mold on a cookie sheet . add 2 drops of your favorite essential oil into the middle inside each mould.

5. Then, add the melted cocoa butter and the lavender tea mixture in the mold.

6. Let the bath melt cool, and then place it placed in the freezer to cool for about 20 minutes.

7. Take the bath melts off the silicon tray and take a bath. the relaxing bath.

PART 2

BATH BOMB RECIPES

If you are making bath bombs, don't be intimidated by the lack of molds as you do not require any specific equipment to make your bombs. There are a myriad of items which can be utilized in the making of bath bombs. For instance, a 2-part Christmas ornament that snaps together is a handy mold which could be utilized to create circles of bath bombs from home. You can purchase the mold from craft stores, and If you're not able to find one, just mold your bombs into balls using your hands.

There are many items that work well as molds that are improvised. For example, when creating round bombs, molds could be created by cut of tennis balls into half.

Some other examples are ice-cube tray, muffin trays, shot glasses, etc.

In general, it's simpler to create smaller bath bombs since larger ones tend to break down, while smaller ones appear to be more durable.

How to make bath bombs

* When you are making your bath bombs, begin with small batches until your ability to know the procedure creating bath bombs. It is possible to begin by making two bath bombs for each batch by reducing the recipe to 2/3 cup baking soda and the 1/3 cup citric acid all at once.

Be sure to wear gloves when you make bath bombs or different bath items.

* Purchase a bowl to mix the citric acid with the baking soda. Make sure that these elements are properly mixed mixing them back and forth using two bowls.

When you're using oils that are essential add them to the mix and mix quickly using your hands prior to when the mixture starts to pop. Be aware that food coloring could make the mix somewhat lumpy, but the clump can be removed by rubbing them in your hands.

* When mixing mix, spray witch hazel or water on the mix each time you mix with only a small amount. Try to achieve consistency during the mixing process until it is able to hold tightly when you squeezed it with your hands.

* Use molds for packing the mixture in a tight. If you're using two-part molds, such as the Christmas decorations It is recommended to fill each portion of your mold slightly filled and then press them together in a tight manner. Do not twist or press when you are removing the bath bomb out of it by tapping it against the mold.

* After that, let the bath bombs in the sun for about two hours. It is important to shield them from the direct sunlight.

Don't put your bath bombs out of the way for too long since they diminish their fizz after a short time. They must have been used in the first couple of weeks after their production. And the earlier they're utilized, the more you will be able to take a aromatic and relaxing bath.

Soothing Bath Bombs in Multi-Color

The bath bombs are vibrant and sparkling. They will give you a sparkling flash of color after you drop one into water.

Ingredients

* 3 cups baking soda

1. 1/2 cup of cornstarch

1. 1/2 cup of citric acid

6. 6 tablespoons coconut oil melt

* Twenty drops essential rose oils

*20 drops Geranium essential oils

* Pink, purple blue, green and yellow mica powder

Two tablespoons of polysorbate 80

* White or silver cosmetic glitter

The Witch Hazel and the rubbing alcohol can be found can be found in the form of a spray bottle

* Poop molds for unicorns

Instructions

* Mix citric soda baking soda, citric acid, and cornstarch to the large mixing bowl. Mix thoroughly to mix the ingredients.

* Add the coconut oil and polysorbate 80 to mix well.

Add essential oils to the mix. Mix it and add the witch hazel or rubbing alcohol to dampen the mix until it resembles the texture of wet sand. Be sure that it is held tightly when you squeeze a few handfuls.

• Divide them equally in five bowls. Add the yellow, green blue, pink and purple micas in the five containers that are smaller and mix well.

* Place the glitter in the mold's cavity. Begin to layer each color in the mold's

cavity and press them firmly inside the mold. Repeat the process for all colors. If the mixture inside the bowls gets dry when pouring it into the molds it with a small amount of alcohol or witch hazel to dampen them.

* Allow the bath bombs in the refrigerator overnight to set. Place a large plate or cutting board over the mold, then flip it to allow the unicorn's bathtub to slip through the hole.

The bath bombs are now ready for use. Place your bath bombs inside an airtight container.

Headache Relief Bath Bombs

These bath bombs aid in helping to ease headaches. They are made from essential oils of peppermint and lavender which are generally used for relaxation and tension relief.

Ingredients

* 1 cup baking soda

1./8 cups of Epsom salts

1. 1/4 Cup of Cornstarch

1/8 of a cup SLSA

* 1 teaspoon of citric acid

1. 1/4 Cup of lavender dried

* 1/2 teaspoon of polysorbate 80

Three tablespoons coconut oil

Ten drops lavender ginger, frankincense, peppermint and chamomile essential oils

* Teal and purple mica powder

* Bath bomb molds

Instructions

* Mix all the baking soda and cornstarch citric acid Epsom salts SLSA and dried lavender in an enormous bowl and mix well (you might require a masks to avoid breathing in SLSA).

* Melt coconut oil with the help of a microwave. Allow it to cool. Add essential

oils and polysorbates 80. Mix the ingredients well.

Include the liquid ingredients into the bowl large enough to hold the dry ingredients. Stir well using your hands and gloves on. Make sure you mix the ingredients thoroughly until you get a smooth texture that resembles wet sand. If the mix isn't pliable and holds tightly when squeezed it then add additional coconut oil. Start by adding one teaspoon at a go and blend it in thoroughly until your desired consistency is achieved.

Make sure you divide your mix into two bowls. Add 1/2 teaspoon of purple mica powder into one bowl, while adding the teal mica in the second bowl. Mix both bowls thoroughly.

* If you would like that your bathing bombs appear to have the appearance of a dark shade You can get this done through adding mica however, be aware that if the mica content is too high it could make the tub dirty.

Start filling the molds with the mix as you pack each addition. Then, press the mixture in the molds.

Then, put the two sides of the mold together and then wipe each edge of the mold to ensure that the edges are sealed. Fill the remainder of the molds and repeat the steps above.

* Tap the molds' ends with a gentle tap and then pop them out. Allow them to dry for at least 24 hours.

* Place in an air tight container.

Revitalizing Charcoal Bath Bombs

These bathing bombs made of charcoal work for cleansing the skin and getting rid of excess oil on the skin. The ingredients used in the making of these bath bombs can be found below.

Ingredients

* 1/4 cup citric acid

* 1/2 cup baking soda

* 2 tbsp. of activated charcoal, food grade

*30 drops essential Frankincense oil

* 6 tbsp. of coconut oil and melted

• A spray bottle with witch hazel

* Bath bomb molds

Instructions

* Take baking sodaand charcoal and citric acid mixed together in an enormous glass bowl.

* The coconut oil should be melted and let it cool. Mix it with the other dry components. Add the essential oil and mix well.

Make sure the mixture has the same texture as wet sand. it is able to hold together when you squeeze a few handfuls. If it isn't holding it, lightly spray the mixture with witch hazel, and mix thoroughly.

Begin filling the part of the mold and making sure to pack each addition carefully. The second side that is filled just a bit more than its top so that it creates a small dome.

Then press the two halves together with a firm press and then wipe all edges, making sure the two sides are properly sealed. Repeat the process until are finished with the mix.

* Lastly, take the bath bombs from the molds, and allow the bath bombs to air dry for approximately 24 hours.

Lifting Orange Bath Bombs

These bath bombs are delightful. They smell of orange and come with a range of benefits. These include relaxation for the mind and body as well as nourishment for the skin.

Ingredients

* 2 cups baking soda

1 cup Epsom salt

1. 1 Cup of Cornstarch

1. 1 Cup of citric acid

* 20 drops of essential orange oil

* 1/4 cup almond oil

• A spray bottle that contains witch hazel

* Mica or body glitter for glitz (optional)

* Orange gel food coloring

* Bath bomb molds

Instructions

* Put all the dry ingredients in large bowls and mix them well.

Mix the wet ingredients in a separate bowl. Then, mix the wet ingredients and the dry ingredients, making sure that they are well blended. Sprinkle the mixture with witch hazel, and mix until you have the consistency of sand that is damp.

* If you're using glitter or mica, you can sprinkle them on the molds prior to placing the bath bomb mix inside the molds. Put the mixture in moulds, until they are overfilled.

* After that you can join the two halves tightly and allow them to dry over the course of the night.

• Remove the bombs out of the molds and place them inside an airtight container, or put them in shrink wrap bags so that they keep their scent.

A refreshing lemon Bath Bombs

These amazing bath bombs have the fresh scent of vanilla and lemon. The skin is left feeling soft and soft.

Ingredients

* 3 cups baking soda

34 cup Epsom salts

1. 1/2 cup of citric acid

1. 1/2 cup of cornstarch

* Food coloring of yellow

* 15 drops essential lemon oil

* 15 drops of vanilla essential oil

* 1/4 cup coconut oil and melt it

• A spray bottle that contains witch hazel

* Bath bomb molds

Instructions

Mix together your baking soda, citric acid cornstarch as well as Epsom salts in one big bowl.

Add the melted coconut oil to the mix and stir thoroughly. After that, lightly spray with witch hazel, and mix until you have that consistency you would expect from wet sandy.

Divide the mixture in two bowls using a measuring 1/3 in one bowl and 2/3 in the second bowl.

Incorporate vanilla essential oil into the smaller batch, and mix lemon essential oil along with some of the yellow coloring in the second batch. Make sure to mix thoroughly.

* Put the lemon and vanilla bath bombs in layers of roughness into the half-molds.

Then, press the mixture into the molds until slightly full.

* Make sure you press the two mold halves tightly and then leave them for a couple of minutes.

* Remove the bombs from the molds , and let them dry for 24 hours prior to use.

Invigorating coffee bath bombs

These gorgeous bath bombs smell of coffee. They also aid in increasing blood flow in the body, as well as improving energy levels.

Ingredients

• 3/4 cup powdered dry milk

1. 1/2 cup of citric acid

* 3 cups baking soda

* 6 tablespoons instant espresso powder

2 tablespoons of Jojoba coconut or jojoba

Spray bottle that contains witch hazel

* Bath bomb molds

Instructions

* Combine all the dry ingredients together in a container, then mix. Add oil and mix until it is well blended.

Make sure that the mix is the same as what you would expect from wet sand, and it stays together when you squeeze a few handfuls. If it doesn't it, lightly spray the mixture with witch hazel, and mix thoroughly.

* Fill the molds with the mix while taking care with each addition. Then, press the mixture inside the molds.

* Put the two halves of the molds tightly and then wipe each mold's edges, making sure that the sides have been sealed. Fill in the remainder of the molds by repeating the steps above.

* Lastly, take the bath bombs out of the molds and allow them to dry for around 24 hours.

Relaxing Vanilla Bath Bombs

The bathing bombs ideal to relax at evening in the bath. They can be used for relaxing of the mind as well as the skin.

Ingredients

* 3 cups baking soda

1. 1/2 cup of Epsom salt

1. 1/2 cup of citric acid

*30 drops essential oil of chamomile

* 3 tsp. of vanilla extract

Spray bottle with witch hazel

* 2 tbsp. of sweet olive oil or almond oil

* 3 tsp. of dried lavender buds

* Bath bomb molds

Instructions

* Mix baking soda, citric acid and lavender buds to an empty bowl and whisk them all together.

Mix olive oil, essential oil along with vanilla extract into an additional bowl.

Include the wet ingredient into the dry ingredients in the bowl Mix them quickly using your hands (with gloves put on).

Make sure the mixture is comparable to that of wet sand. it stays together by squeezing a small amount. If it doesn't it, lightly spray the mixture with witch hazel, and mix thoroughly.

The molds should be filled with the mix, making sure to pack each addition carefully. Then, press the mixture inside the molds.

* Put the two parts of the mold in a firmly and clean each edge of the mold, making sure both sides have been sealed. Fill in the remainder of the molds, repeating the steps above.

* Lastly, remove your bathing bombs out of the mold and let their drying for approximately 24 hours.

Hydrating Butterscotch Bath Bombs

These bath bombs provide an aroma of sweet butterscotch. They're soothing and good for skin.

Ingredients

* 3 cups baking soda

1. 1/2 cup of Epsom salt

1. 1/2 tablespoons bronze and gold cosmetic pigment powder

1. 1/2 cup of cornstarch

* 1/2 cup citric acid

• A spray bottle with witch hazel

*20 drops butterscotch oils

*30 drops grape seed essential oil

* Bath bomb molds

Instructions

Blend baking soda Epsom salt, cornstarch and citric acid in an enormous bowl.

Divide the mixture into two bowls. Add the cosmetic color Start with around 1 teaspoon, and then increase until you achieve the desired color.

Mix the grapeseed oil and butterscotch scent in a small bowl and mix it all to mix. Mix the liquid in each bowl and mix vigorously to ensure that the mix doesn't get activated.

Make sure the mixture is comparable in consistency to wet sand and holds by squeezing a small amount. If it doesn't it, lightly spray the mixture with witch hazel, and mix thoroughly.

* The bath bomb mix should be layered into the molds and alternate the bronze and the gold. Then press it hard in the molds.

Then, put the two sides of the mold together and clean each edge of the mold to ensure that the sides have been sealed. Fill in the rest of the molds, repeating the steps above.

* Finally, take your bathing bombs out of the mold and let the bath bombs to air dry for approximately 24 hours.

Hot Relief Bath Bombs

The bath bombs can be created using VapoRub to aid in the relaxation of muscles and clear sinuses in the cold season.

Ingredients

Two cups corn starch

* 6 tbsp. of VapoRub

* 4 tbsp. of water

* Blue and green soap colorant

Instructions

* Add VapoRub into a bowl. You can make any kind of vapor rub that you like.

* Add corn starch , and stir until the ingredients are blended. Add 2 tablespoons of water, and stir until you have a smooth mixture.

• Add one drop blue and green soap coloring. Mix well to mix.

* Take a few ounces of the mix and then knead it into an oval. Place the balls on the wax paper. Then let them dry.

Fresh Herbal Bath Bombs

The bath bombs are refreshing and herbal. They are made from herbs that relax the body and provide nourishment to the skin.

Ingredients

6. 6 tablespoons dried lavender flowers

• 3/4 cups of calendula flowers that have been dried

* 1/4 cup dried Chamomile flower

*30 drops Roman ou lavender essential oils

* 1/2 cup of herbs almond oil

Half cup Epsom salt

1. 1 Cup of Cornstarch

* 3 cups baking soda

* 1/2 cup citric acid

Spray bottle that contains witch hazel

* Bath bomb molds

Instructions

Blend all the herbs that you have dried in your blender. blend with the remaining of the dried herbs in a bowl.

Mix almond oil and essential oils in a separate bowl. Slowly add the wet mix to the container large enough to hold dried ingredients. Be careful not to pour it in too fast , as it could ruin the batch.

Make sure the mixture is comparable to what you would expect from wet sand, and it is able to hold together by squeezing a small amount. If it isn't it, lightly spray the mixture with witch hazel, and mix thoroughly.

* Fill the molds with the mix while making sure to pack each addition carefully. Make sure to press it in the molds.

* Put the two parts of the mold in a firmly and then wipe each edge of the mold to ensure that the sides have been sealed. Fill the remainder of the molds and repeat the process above.

• Finally, take out all bath bombs that have mold, and allow the bath bombs to air dry for approximately 24 hours.

Fortifying Spiced Pumpkin Bath Bombs

This is the perfect bath bomb recipe that is perfect for autumn time. They are gorgeous and, when they come in contact with water they change to a stunning orange.

Ingredients

34 cup Epsom salts

1. 1 Cup of Corn Starch

1. 1/2 cup of citric acid

* 3 cups baking soda

*40 drops pumpkin pie scent

* 3 tsp. from pumpkin pie spices, with additional decorations

* Orange gel dye

* 3 tbsp. of coconut oil melting

Spray bottle that contains witch hazel

Instructions

* Mix all dry ingredients together in one large bowl, and combine thoroughly. Add essential oils and coconut oil that has been melted and mix until it is well-mixed.

* Stir 8-10 drops of Orange gel dye to the mix. Be sure the dye is evenly distributed. You can also sprinkle a few drops of witch hazel if you need.

Make sure the mixture is comparable in consistency to wet sand and holds when you squeeze a few handfuls. If it isn't holding then lightly spray the mix with witch hazel, and mix thoroughly.

Sprinkle the molds with a bit of cinnamon and pumpkin pie. Fill the molds up with the mixture , making sure to pack each one carefully. Then, press it in the molds.

* Put the two sides of the mold in a firmly and clean each edge of the mold, making sure that the edges are sealed. Fill in the rest of the molds, repeating the steps above.

* Lastly, take all bath bombs that have mold and let their drying for approximately 24 hours.

The exotic Doughnut Bath Bombs

The gorgeous bath bombs can be handed out as gifts to your loved ones and relatives. The bombs are simple to make.

Ingredients

Half cup Epsom salt

* 1/2 cup corn starch

* 1/2 cup citric acid

* 3 cups baking soda

Colors: Pink Cosmetic Grade

* Sprinkles

* 1 lb. of goat's milk soap that has been melted to form a base

*30 drops of essential oils, such as orange or lavender.

Three tablespoons of coconut oil melting

• A spray bottle with witch hazel

* Donut bath bomb molds

Instructions

Mix the baking soda, citric acid and cornstarch Epsom salt and the pigment in a large bowl.

Blend the oil essential and the coconut oil that is melted in the container of a small size. Add other dry ingredients, mixing until well blended.

Make sure the mixture is comparable in consistency to wet sand and that it stays together when you squeeze a few handfuls. If it isn't holding it, lightly spray the mixture with witch hazel, and mix thoroughly.

* Fill the molds with the mix, making sure to pack each addition carefully. Make sure to press it inside the molds.

Then, put the two parts of the mold in a firmly and then wipe each edge of the mold to ensure both edges are sealed. Fill the remainder of the molds and repeat the steps above.

* Let the bath bombs air dry within the mold around 24 hours.

* Melt the base of milk soap and then drip it over the bath bombs that are donuts after they have been dry. Add sprinkles as soon as you can and let the soap sit for around 10 minutes.

Delightful Candy Corn Bath Bombs

These bath bombs work great to give as gifts, particularly during the autumn months such as Halloween. Ingredients used in making these bath bomb sets are listed below.

Ingredients

3 cups of cornstarch

* 1/2 cup citric acid

* 3 cups baking soda

* 1/4 cup coconut oil

14 cup SLSA

* 1 1/2 tbsp. of polysorbate 80

* The fragrance of candy corn

Spray bottle with witch hazel

* Glitter (optional)

* White pearl, yellow along with orange, mica

* Bath bomb molds

Instructions

* Add baking soda cornstarch, and citric soda along with the SLSA in the big mixing bowl.

You can add coconut oil as well as candy corn fragrance and polysorbate 80 and mix it until well combined.

The mixture should be divided in three bowls. Include white pearl mica in one bowl and yellow mica to another bowl and orange mica to another bowl. Mix the contents of both bowls until they are the mixture is well-mixed.

* Make sure that the mix is comparable in consistency to wet sand and that it stays together by squeezing a small amount. If it isn't holding it, lightly spray the mixture with witch hazel, and mix thoroughly.

* Purchase a bath bomb mold, and then fill up the first part of the mold up to 1/4 of the way full with the white mixture , then pat it lightly. Fill it up with orange, then make sure that the yellow is added to the second half of the mold until about 2/3. Then, press it in the mold. The remaining portion part of the mold using the mixture of orange.

* Put the two sides of the mold together and then wipe all edges to ensure that the sides have been sealed. Fill in the

remainder of the molds and repeat the steps above.

* Let the bath bombs remain in molds to dry for approximately 24 hours.

Sweet Strawberry Bath Bombs

These bath bombs are simple to make and have the most delicious strawberry fragrance. The ingredients that are used to make these bath bomb sets are listed below.

Ingredients

1.1/2 cups citric acid

*1 cup corn starch

* 3 cups baking soda

• 1 Cup Epsom salts

* 6 tbsp. of strawberry powder

* 4 tsp. from strawberry fragrance oil

* 6 tbsp. of almond oil

Spray bottle that contains witch hazel

* Bath bomb molds

Instructions

* Put Epsom salts, baking soda, citric acid corn starch and strawberry powder into one large bowl. Mix until combined.

Mix both almond and strawberry fragrance oils in a tiny container.

Mix the wet and dry ingredients, and mix until they are well-combined.

Make sure the mixture is comparable as the texture of wet sand and holds when you squeeze a few handfuls. If it doesn't then lightly spray the mix with witch hazel, and mix thoroughly.

Fill the molds as you pack each addition. Then, press the mixture inside the molds.

Then, put the two parts of the mold in a firmly and clean any edges, making sure that the sides are properly sealed.

* Let the bath bombs air dry within the molds around 24 hours.

Rejuvenating Mermaid Bath Bombs

These bath bombs are packed with vibrant sprinkles that easily dissolve in the water. They make the perfect gift to your those you love dearly.

Ingredients

* 1 cup cream from tartar

* 1/2 Cups of SLSA

1. 1/2 cup of citric acid

* 3 cups baking soda

*20 drops essential grapefruit oil

* 20 drops of lime essential oil or essential oil of orange

Spray bottle with witch hazel

* 6 tbsp. of coconut oil melting

* Mermaid inspired sprinkles

* Bath bomb molds

* Red, blue,, and turquoise micas.

Instructions

* Mix baking soda, citric acid SLSA as well as cream of tartar in the large mixing bowl, and mix thoroughly.

* Make sure all lumps of the dry mixture are broken before moving into the following step.

* In an ice cube to mix the coconut oil with essential oils.

Mix the ingredients in the liquids with the dry ones gradually and mix well until the liquid is well integrated to the dry mixture.

The mixture should be divided to three small bowls equally. Add blue mica powder to one of the bowls. Then, add the purple mica powder to the second and pink mica to another bowl. Mix the contents in each bowl until it is combined.

Make sure the mixture is comparable as the texture of wet sand and holds by squeezing a handful. If it isn't holding then lightly spray the mix with witch hazel, and mix thoroughly.

Fill each mold Mermaid sprinkles. The three colors are placed over the sprinkles inside the mold. Make sure to press them tightly in the molds.

Then, put the two parts of the mold in a firmly and clean each edge of the mold to ensure both edges are covered. Fill the remainder of the molds and repeat the steps above.

* Let the bath bombs remain in molds for approximately 24 hours.

Soothing Bath Bombs for Dinosaurs

These cute bath bombs are ideal for children. The bombs are infused with lavender essential oil, which is known to help calm the body.

Ingredients

* 3/4 cup Epsom salt

* 1/2 cup citric acid

1. 1/2 cup cornstarch

* 3 cups baking soda

* 30 drops lavender oil or essential oil of chamomile

* Natural coloring you like

* Mini Easter egg molds and dinosaurs

• A spray bottle with witch hazel

Instructions

* Mix baking soda, cornstarch along with critic acid into a container, and mix to combine. Add essential oil and color to the mix and mix thoroughly.

* Spray the mixture lightly with witch hazel before mixing. The mix should be like that of fresh sand and it stays together when you squeeze it into a small amount. If it doesn't it, lightly spray the mix with witch hazel, and mix thoroughly.

Begin with filling up the mini dinosaur molds with the mix while taking care with each addition. Then, press it firmly into the molds.

* Let the bath bombs remain in molds for approximately 24 hours.

Calming Snowman Bath Bombs

This is an ideal recipe for bath bombs that is suitable for use in winter. The bath bombs are customizable by using different colors and scents.

Ingredients

1. 1/2 Cup of Cornstarch

Half cup Epsom salt

* 1 Cup of acidic citric

* 1 cup baking soda

* 1/2 tsp. of powdered orange mica

* 1/2 tsp. of charcoal activated powder

* 1/4 tsp. of ruby alcohol

Ten to 20 drops essential oil or fragrance

* 3 tbsp. of coconut oil that is melted

Spray bottle that contains witch hazel

* Bath bomb molds

Instructions

* Combine baking soda, citric acid Epsom salt and cornstarch into one large bowl, and mix well.

Combine coconut oil with essential oil in one small bowl.

Mix the wet ingredients and dry ingredients with care. Make sure the mixture is similar as the texture of wet sand and it stays together when you squeeze it with a spoon. If it isn't it, lightly spray the mixture with witch hazel, and mix thoroughly.

The molds should be filled with the mix, taking care with each addition. Then, press the mixture in the molds.

Then, put the two parts of the mold together and then wipe all edges to ensure both sides have been sealed. Fill in the rest of the molds and repeat the steps above.

* Let the bath bombs remain in molds for approximately 24 hours.

To create the snowman's face, mix some charcoal powder and rubbing alcohol in the ratio of 2:1. Utilizing a paintbrush, add charcoal dots of black into the bombs in order to make the facial features. Repeat the process with the mica that is orange to create that snowman's carrot-like nose.

Drying time is important, then your bath bomb is ready to use.

BATH MELT RECIPES

Bath melts are small bars made from moisturizing body butter that melts when placed in the hot tub. They release a lovely scent and provide a softening skin bathing experience. The butter and oils that are skin-friendly help to moisturise and nourish the skin. Bath melts are made using butters, such as mango butter, cocoa butter and shea butter which are beneficial for the skin.

Bath melts can help reduce stress while bathing. The skin-nourishing oils and fats aid in softening the skin. To provide a more enjoyable and luxurious experience, add dried essential oils and herbs when making your bath melts. However, you must be extra cautious when you get in or out of your tub as the butter and oils that are made into melts can make your tub extremely slippery.

Essential tips for making bath melts

When you make your bath melts, be sure to follow these precautions;

Be sure to wear gloves to safeguard your hands from the heat of the butter and oils melt very hot.

It is important to ensure that the molds that you're using for bath melts are able to take the temperatures. Molds made of silicone are recommended due to of their ability to regulate the temperature to around 500 degrees F.

Place your molds on the cookie sheet or cutting board for help to stabilize it. It makes it much easier to move the molds relocated if needed.

* Make use of dried herbs to stop moisture from becoming trapped in the butter and causing the appearance of a moldy mess.

* Make sure that the molds aren't too big You can also use Ice cube tray.

* To make use of, fill your bathtub with warm water and add a couple of bath melts. Enjoy the bath and relax.

Moisturizing Herbal Bath Melts

These gorgeous bath melts include nutritious butter along with oils wonderful for skin.

Ingredients

1. 1/2 cup dry (lavender roses, lavender or other skin-safe plants)

Two teaspoons sunflower oil or Jojoba oil

* 30 drops of essential rosemary oils

2. teaspoons beeswax grated

1 cup shea butter

1. 1/2 Cup of Cocoa Butter

* Silicone molds

Instructions

• Melt the honey as well as the butter by using two boilers. Let it cool.

* Add the essential oil and sunflower oil and stir well until everything is well mixed.

Set your molds up on the cutting board or cookie sheet. Add dried herbs to each mold.

Then, pour the butter mix over the herb mixture, ensuring it is at fill the entire cavity. Let it cool and set in the refrigerator.

If your bath melts seem too soft then melt them again and add additional wax. Remove them from the molds once they've cooled and place them in glass jars.

Calming Chamomile Bath Melts

These bath melts can nourish your skin while you relax in the bath. They're made of chamomile, which aid in relaxing the body and smooth the skin. This recipe makes use of clove essential oil a scent that offers a wonderful refreshing aroma.

Ingredients

* 1 tbsp. of almond sweet oil

*20 drops essential clove oil

1. 1 Cup of Shea Butter

* 1 tbsp. in white pasteilles

* 1 tbsp. of dried flowers of chamomile

* Clamshell containers

Instructions

* Melt your beeswax and shea butter by using Double boiler methods. Allow it to cool.

• Add the sweet almond oil as well as essential oils and mix until it is a blend.

* Pour the mixture in the clamshell containers , but don't overfill them. make sure to leave room for flowers of chamomile.

• Add flowers, and then put the bath melts in the refrigerator for around 30 minutes.

* Pull out the bath melts from the refrigerator and take them out of the containers in clamshells.

Fortifying Chocolate Bath Melts

The amazing bath melts contain the heavenly chocolate scent of the herb cocoa powder that adds a delicious scent. In addition to the smell of chocolate, they're made from cosmetic oils and butter, which can be beneficial for skin. They can hydrate the skin, nourish it, and soften your skin.

Ingredients

* 1/2 tsp. of cocoa powder made from organic cocoa

* 1 tsp. of white pastilles made of beeswax

1. 1/2 Cup of Cocoa Butter

Shea Butter 1/4 Cup

1. 1/4 Cup of mango butter

* 15 drops essential oil of frankincense

* Ice cube tray

Instructions

* Melt the butter and beeswax by using Double boiler methods. Let it cool and then add the cocoa powder and mix it vigorously to mix it.

* Add the essential oil and mix to combine.

* Pour the mix into the tray of ice cubes and put it in the fridge or let it dry in a dry, cool location.

* Pull out your bath melts once they have cooled and then store them in a dry, cool area.

Relaxing Lavender Bath Melts

The moisturizing bath melts come with the scent of a relaxing and soothing that can aid in relaxation and boosts energy. They also provide nourishment to your skin, leaving it silky and soft.

Ingredients

* 2 tbsp. of dried lavender flowers

* 1 tsp. of white pastilles made of beeswax

* 1 tbsp. of sunflower oil

1. 1 Cup of Cocoa Butter

Ten drops Geranium essential oil

Ten drops essential oil of lavender

* Clamshell containers

Instructions

* Melt the cocoa butter and beeswax using the double boiler method.

* Add essential oil and sunflower oil to the mix and mix until it is well blended.

* Pour the mixture into clamshells slowly and leave space for the calendula blooms.

Sprinkle the flowers over the mix and place the bath to melt inside the refrigerator once it's cool.

Take fridge out after it has cooled and place in a cool dry area.

Moisture-Rich Pumpkin Bath Melts

These nourishing bath melts are shaped in the shape of cute pumpkins. They are as a nice decoration for the holiday season of thanksgiving and Halloween. The beautiful mica dust is used as a decoration to make bath melts a gorgeous sparkle. The ingredients that nourish the skin in this recipe renew and nourish the skin.

Ingredients

* 1/2 tsp. from pumpkin spice mix powder

* 1/2 tsp. from pumpkin seed powder

* 1 tbsp. of oil extracted from pumpkin seeds

* 1 tsp. of white pastilles of beeswax

1 cup cocoa butter

1. 1/4 Cup of mango butter

1 cup palm oil

• 20 drops essential grapefruit oil

* 1/4 tsp. of gold mica

* 1/4 tsp. of mica dust diamond

* 24 mini pumpkins Silicone soap mold

Instructions

• Melt butters, honey and oils by using two boilers. Allow the mixture to cool.

* Include the essential oil, spice blend for pumpkin pie, along with the diamond and gold micas.

* Pour the mix into the mold made of silicone.

* Cool, then put in the refrigerator to set.

Take the refrigerator out and keep in a dry, cool area.

Relaxing Bath Melts of Roses

The bath melts come with an uplifting fragrance. The gorgeous pink rose petals that are used in this recipe can boost your mood thanks to its subtle scent.

Ingredients

* 1/2 tsp. of powdered beetroot

* 1 tsp. of white pastilles made of beeswax

1 cup cocoa butter

1 cup mango butter

1 cup shea butter

• 20 drops essential jasmine oil

* Pink rose petals

• 24 miniature hearts in silicone soap mold

Instructions

The butters can be melted and the the beeswax with two boilers. Let it cool slightly.

* Mix in the powder of beetroot and mix quickly using a stick or spoon until the ingredients are mixed. Include the oil of fragrance, and stir to combine.

* Pour the batter into molds, then sprinkle the herbs evenly over the batter inside each mold. Cool and then place them in the fridge to firm up.

* Take the bath melts out of the mold and keep them in a dry, cool area.

Uplifting Jasmine Bath Melts

These bath melts are ideal to relax in the tub and can help improve your mood and nourish the skin. The recipe makes use of Cocoa Butter and coconut oil, which provides nourishment and hydration to the skin.

Ingredients

* 1 tbsp. of rosebuds and petals

* 1 tsp. of white pastilles made of beeswax

* 1/3 cup coconut oil

3 cups of cocoa butter

*20 drops essential jasmine oil

* Ice cube tray

Instructions

* Melt your coconut oil, cocoa butter along with the beeswax using your double boiler. Let the mixture cool slightly.

* Add the essential jasmine oil to the mix, and stir well to combine.

Pour the mix into the tray of ice cubes Make sure to leave room for petals and rosebuds.

* Sprinkle petals and rosebuds on the mix, then put it in the refrigerator to set.

Take the refrigerator out and place in a dry, cool area.

The Bath Melts that stimulate parsley are a great way to do this.

This recipe for a bath melt makes use of substances that nourish and soothe the skin. This recipe for bath and body is scented with a pleasant aroma that can be used to relax and can help you get the rest of your night.

Ingredients

* 1/2 tsp. of powdered parsley leaves

* 1 tsp. of pastilles of white beeswax

1 cup cocoa butter

1 cup mango butter

Shea Butter 1/4 Cup

Ten drops essential lavender oil

* 10 drops essential rose oil

* Pink rose petals

• 24 miniature hearts made of silicone soap molds

Instructions

Make sure to melt your beeswax, butters, and butters by using Double boiler methods. Allow it to cool.

* Add the powdered parsley leaves into the mixture and stir it vigorously.

Incorporate the essential oil, and stir to mix the mix.

Pour the mix in the silicone mini hearts molds, then sprinkle with flowers of the pink variety.

* Put them in the fridge to set. Remove the fridge from the freezer and remove the molds.

* Keep it in a dry, cool area.

Luxury white chocolate bath melts

This recipe is made with white chocolate, which is known for its ability to nourish your skin. The bath melts will provide you with a the most delicious scent that is refreshing. Ingredients

Five white chocolate wafers

* 1 tbsp. of white pastilles of beeswax

1-cup mango butter

* 1 tbsp. of Apricot kernel oil (optional)

* 1-2 tsp. of fragrance oil white chocolate

* 24 bites of brown soap molds made from silicone

Instructions

Then, melt the beeswax, butter as well as white chocolate, by using Double boiler technique. Let cool.

* Add the fragrance oil of white chocolate and apricot kernel oils (if you are using). Stir until the mixture is well blended.

* Pour the batter into the molds for brownie bites made from silicone.

* Cool before placing melting baths inside the freezer to set.

* Take the mold out of the refrigerator after it has cooled, remove it of the mold and keep in a dry, cool location.

Revitalizing Lavender Lemon Bath Melts

These bath melts are ideal to smooth your skin. The healthy herbs in this recipe provide the bath melts an enchanting smell.

Ingredients

* Lavender buds

* 1/2 tsp. lemon peel powder

* 1 tsp. from white pastilles made of beeswax

1. 1/2 Cup of Cocoa Butter

1 cup mango butter

Shea Butter 1/4 Cup

* 10 drops lavender essential oil

* 10 drops lemon essential oil

* Silicone molds or an ice cube tray

Instructions

* Melt butters and beeswax by using two boilers. Let it cool.

* Add the powder of the lemon peel and mix with a spoon to make a complete mix. Add essential oils and mix.

* Pour the mix into the molds and then sprinkle the molds with lavender flowers.

* Place in the refrigerator to set. Remove the molds from the refrigerator once the molds are solid. Remove the molds from the refrigerator and place in a dry, cool area.

Healing Calendula Bath Melts

This wonderful recipe for bath melts includes calendula flower petals an incredible herb that works to reduce acne and inflammation.

Ingredients

* 2 tsp. of grape seed oil

1. 1 Cup of Mango Butter

* 1 tbsp. of white pastilles made of beeswax

* 2 tsp. from calendula flowers

* Sandalwood essential oil

* Clamshell containers

Instructions

The mango butter is melted and the beeswax using this double boiler technique. Let it cool.

* Add grapeseed oil and sandalwood essential oil , and mix to mix.

* Put the mix into the clamshells cautiously, while leaving enough room for the calendula flower.

* Sprinkle the calendula flower onto each of the clamshells. After that, you can press the petals in the melt of your bath with care.

The bath melts should be placed in the refrigerator to set. Remove the bath melts from the fridge once the bath melts are solid.

* Take the molds out of the molds, and keep them in a dry, cool area.

BATH TRUFFFLE RECIPES

Bath truffles consist of tiny fizz since they are made from the citric acid as well as sodium bicarbonate. As opposed to regular bombs they are believed to be more emollient due to the fact that they contain more butter. The equipment needed to make bath truffles comprise the following:

• Large mixing bowl

* Kitchen scales

* The right molds will be needed to form the truffles in the bath, but this is not required since you are able to employ your hands to form your truffles.

The most common ingredients required for bath truffles are the following:

* Citric acid
* Cocoa butter or Shea butter
* Baking soda
* Polysorbate-80
* Essential oils and scent oils of your choice
* Dry flower petals, or cosmetic glitter that is an option
* Food coloring, though not mandatory is also available.

General instructions for making bath truffles

If you have all the equipment and ingredients in your kitchen Follow the steps below to make your bath truffles

i. By using a double boiler melt the shea butter slowly.

ii. When it is completely turned into liquid, take it off the heat and add polysorbate-

80. Mix the ingredients and allow to cool a little.

iii. Add essential oils to mix after it has been allowed to it is cool, and mix.

iv. Measure the baking soda, as well as the critic acid into an mixing bowl. If necessary, sieve and mix them until they are well blended.

V. If you wish to use a powdered color in the future, you should add a tiny amount at a moment until your desired shade is created.

vi. Incorporate the liquid ingredients into the dry components, and mix the dough until it is well-mixed.

vii. It is crucial to include enough shea butter into the truffle, so that when you hold it and squeeze only a tiny amount it retains its shape. A slightly oily surface can appear, making it crucial. But, you must make sure that the mixture does not contain excess oil than what is needed to get it well-compressed.

viii. You can put a tiny amount of the mixture and place it in the palms of your hands and make it into the shape of a ball. It is also possible to get the mix pressed into silicone or plastic mold.

ix. After you have a solid ball, sprinkle petals or cosmetic glitter on the table or board and then gently roll the bath truffle around in the petals or glitters afterward.

x. Place the truffle onto a greaseproof paper with care and repeat the process until the entire mixture has been utilized.

xi. The truffles should be firm for between forty and sixty minutes. The shea butter will become pretty solid and hard.

xii. Allow them to dry overnight until they are completely hard and then place them in cake cases following to make a beautiful gift If you would like.

xiii. To make use of the product, add a truffle into the bath water or break it to release more bubbles.

Note

* The flower petals may be added to the mix but it may cause the mixture harder to hold together by balls, so don't overdo it.

* Use small cupcake molds or other molds that have a shape to create different shapes than balls.

* If you opt to make use of cocoa butter, keep in mind that the more brittle the texture of the butter, the more difficult the truffles will be due to the butter is not as sticky, and might not hold the petals as well. They are , however, easy to pack as they will not melt when temperatures are low or cause damage to packaging.

Aromatic Cherry Bath Truffles

They smell amazing and easily foam in the tub. The ingredients for this recipe are sure to make your skin feeling soft and soft and.

Ingredients

* 1 cup baking soda

1. 1/2 Cup of SLSA

* 2 tbsp. of Shea butter

14 cup Epsom salt

* 1 Cup of acidic citric

Amount of 20 drops jasmine vital

* 1/8 tsp. Of Neon's Pink Pleasures Powder

1. 1/4 cup Cocoa Butter

* Ice cream scoop

Instructions

* Put baking soda as well as citric acid into an empty bowl. Mix until well-combined.

• Add SLSA (use masks for this procedure to avoid breathing in this powder) and mix thoroughly. Divide the mixture between two bowls.

• Add half the powder of neon pink pleasures in a bowl and mix well. Add essential oil to each bowl, stirring until well-integrated, and finally put aside.

* Melt the cocoa butter and shea butter in the double boiler. Incorporate the butters

that have been melted into the dry ingredient bowls. Use a spatula or a whisk to mix the ingredients.

* Fill half of the scoop with pink mix and the remaining portion with the white mixture.

Place your scoop onto a baking sheet , and keep going until you've used all of the mix.

* Then step is to mix Epsom salt in the rest of the colors. Sprinkle the mix on the truffles in your bath. Allow the truffles to dry overnight.

The Bubbling Raspberry Bath Truffles

These simple bath truffles are stunning. The delicious fragrance oil makes a perfect, bubbly and delicious bath truffle.

Ingredients

* 1 Cup of acidic citric

* 1/2 cup baking soda

* 2 tbsp. of cream of tartar

* 34 cup SLSA

* 1 tbsp. of Polysorbate 80

1/3 cup of Shea Butter

13 cup Cocoa Butter

* 1/2 tbsp. Of Raspberry Jam fragrance oil

* 1 tbsp. from Raspberry seed oil

* 1 1/2 tbsp. of Liquid Glycerin

* 1/4 tsp. of poppy seeds

* 1/2 tsp. of Raspberry mica

Instructions

Then, melt cocoa butter shea butter along with raspberry seed oil with the double boiler.

* Add liquid glycerin polysorbate 80, as well as the fragrance oil to the mix and mix it thoroughly. Set mixture aside.

* In another bowl, thoroughly mix baking soda, citric acid along with cream of tartar.

1. Add SLSA (you might have to wear a mask during this procedure to prevent

breathing in this powder) and then mix the ingredients until well blended.

• Add oil mix in the dry mixture. Utilize your hands to blend all the ingredients (you must wear gloves). Make sure that the ingredients are thoroughly combined.

Divide the mixture into two bowls. Add the mica from the raspberry to one bowl and mix thoroughly. Add the poppy seeds to the second bowl, mixing until well blended.

* Lay a piece of parchment paper over your counter and sprinkle it with baking powder to stop your truffles from joining to each other.

* Spread the pink mixture onto the paper, and make it spread out using your hands to create an oval shape. Put the white dough on the pink mix , and spread it equally to be a perfect match with the pink mix.

CPSIA information can be obtained
at www.ICGtesting.com
Printed in the USA
LVHW040614201222
735554LV00012B/517

9 781998 769438